Menopause

How You Can Benefit from Diet, Vitamins, Minerals, Herbs, Exercise, and Other Natural Methods

Michael T. Murray, N.D.

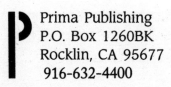
Prima Publishing
P.O. Box 1260BK
Rocklin, CA 95677
916-632-4400

Production by Melanie Field, Bookman Productions
Copyediting by Toni Murray
Typography by ExecuStaff
Interior design by Suzanne Montazer, Bookman Productions
Cover design by The Dunlavey Studio, Sacramento

Library of Congress Cataloging-in-Publication Data

Murray, Michael T.
   Menopause / Michael T. Murray.
     p.   cm. — (Getting well naturally series)
   Includes index.
   ISBN 1-55958-427-0 (pbk.) : $8.95
   1. Menopause—Complications—Alternative treatment.
2. Naturopathy I. Title. II. Series.
RG186.M87 1994
618.1′75—dc20
                                             93-41651
                                               CIP

   95 96 97 98 CWO 10 9 8 7 6 5 4 3
Printed in the United States of America

How to Order:

Single copies may be ordered from Prima Publishing, P.O. Box 1260BK, Rocklin, CA 95677; telephone **916-632-4400.** Quantity discounts are also available. On your letterhead, include information concerning the intended use of the books and the number of books you wish to purchase.

Contents

13   Design of an Exercise Program   159

Preface

Menopause denotes the cessation of menstruation. It usually occurs when a woman reaches the age of 50. A woman is said to have reached menopause if she goes for 6 to 12 months without a period. The time prior to the official designation of menopause is often referred to as perimeno-pausal; the time after menopause is called postmenopause.

According to the current medical view, menopause is more of a disease than a normal physiological process. This view is in stark contrast to the view found in many traditional cultures. People in many other cultures view menopause as a natural part of the life process and a posi-tive event in a woman's life. In fact, in many cultures of the world, most women do not go through the symptoms associated with menopause. This observation raises some interesting questions about the role of culture in the physical experience of menopause.

The current medical view is that menopause has a very negative impact on a woman's life. This view may reflect a male-dominated medical system. Male doctors may not be perceiving accurately how women view menopause.

Studies of women who experience natural menopause have found that women tend to be relieved when menopause occurs, not saddened. In other words, more women view menopause as a positive, rather than a negative, experience.

With the prolongation of life expectancy, the menopausal and postmenopausal periods are becoming more and more significant in a woman's life. In fact, today's average woman can expect to live at least one-third of her life in the postmenopausal phase.

Current medical treatment of menopause primarily involves the use of hormone replacement therapy, which calls for taking a combination of estrogen and progesterone. The obvious question is, Is hormone replacement therapy necessary? The goals of this book are to allow you to answer this question and to provide a natural approach to menopause and the postmenopausal period.

I imagine most women will read this book to find a natural solution to their menopausal symptoms. Such solutions are provided in Section II, but I wanted to provide much more. In Section III, I have provided guidelines that will enable women not to just survive menopause, but to flourish through and beyond it.

Is this possible? Most definitely. Many of the health conditions that afflict postmenopausal women are entirely preventable through proper diet, exercise, and lifestyle. Specifically, natural measures can prevent and sometimes reverse osteoporosis, breast cancer, arthritis, and heart disease.

There is a new paradigm, or model, emerging in medicine. The old paradigm viewed the body as a machine; the new paradigm focuses on the interconnectedness of body, mind, emotions, social factors, and the environment. Rather than relying on drugs and surgery, the new model utilizes natural, noninvasive techniques to promote health and healing.

An interesting aspect of this new paradigm is that it draws from the healing wisdom of many cultures where menopause is viewed in a positive light. The role of the physician or healer in this new paradigm is to facilitate the normal passage into the postmenopausal period by using natural and nontoxic therapies when needed.

My wish for you and for the readers of the other books in the Getting Well Naturally series is that you will follow the recommendations so you can live a healthier life.

Acknowledgments

The major blessings in my life are my family and friends. My love for them truly make lifes worth living.

Special appreciations to my wife, Gina, for being the answer to so many of my dreams; to my parents, Cliff and Patty Murray, and my grandmother, Pauline Shier, for a strong foundation and a lifetime of good memories; to Bob and Kathy Bunton for their love and acceptance; to Ben Dominitz and everyone at Prima for their commitment and support of my work; to Terry Lemerond and everyone at Enzymatic Therapy for all their friendship and support over the years; to Joseph Pizzorno and the students and faculty at Bastyr College who have given me encouragement and support; and finally, I am eternally grateful to all the researchers, physicians, and scientists who over the years have strived to better understand the use of natural medicines. Without their work, this series would not exist, and medical progress would halt.

Michael T. Murray, N.D.
September 1993

Before You Read On

- Do not self-diagnose. Proper medical care is critical to good health. If you have symptoms suggestive of an illness, please consult a physician—preferably a naturopath, holistic physician or osteopath, chiropractor, or other natural health care specialist.
- If you are currently taking a prescription medication, you absolutely must consult your doctor before discontinuing it.
- If you wish to try the natural approach, discuss it with your physician. Since he or she is most likely unaware of the natural alternatives available, you may need to do some educating. Bring this book along with you to the doctor's office. The natural alternatives being recommended are based upon published studies in medical journals. Key references are provided if your physician wants additional information.
- Remember, although many natural alternatives, such as nutritional supplements and plant-based medicines, are effective on their own, they work even better if they are part of a comprehensive natural treatment plan that focuses on diet and lifestyle.

I

Current Views
of Menopause

Chapter 1 will answer the most common question about menopause: Is estrogen replacement therapy necessary? Most women already know, innately, the answer to this question. Unfortunately, they are often swayed by the well-intentioned medical doctor who prescribes estrogen to artificially stimulate menstruation. If you are taking estrogen for this reason, I strongly encourage you to examine the evidence, weigh the risks, and formulate your own opinion about what is best for you.

Chapter 1 will encourage menopausal women to examine the way they view menopause as well as help them choose between the primary alternatives that lie before them: the natural approach and estrogen replacement therapy. If you decide on the natural approach, the remainder of the book will help you develop a successful plan to implement it.

1

Is Estrogen Replacement Therapy Necessary?

By the time most women reach menopause, they are very familiar with the menstrual cycle. The menstrual cycle reflects the monthly rhythmic changes in the secretion rates of the female hormones and corresponding changes in the female organs, including changes in the lining of the uterus.

The menstrual cycle is controlled by the actions of the female hormonal system. Each month during the reproductive years, the secretion of the female hormones is designed to accomplish two primary goals: (1) to ensure that only a single egg is released by the ovaries each month and (2) to prepare the lining of the uterus, the endometrium, for implantation of the fertilized egg. To accomplish these goals, the concentrations of the female sexual hormones fluctuate.

The Female Hormonal System

The ovaries are the major site of manufacture for the female sex hormones, estrogen and progesterone. These hormones are produced by the cells that house eggs (ova), each egg (ovum), inside a follicle. Each month during the reproductive years, the follicle-stimulating hormone (FSH) and luteinizing hormone (LH) secreted by the pituitary cause several follicles to become active and grow. This stimulation causes the active follicles to manufacture estrogen, primarily. When the estrogen level increases to a certain point, conditions are such that, usually, only one follicle bursts and only one egg is released.

After ovulation, what is left of the follicle secretes large quantities of both estrogen and progesterone for about two weeks. After this, if pregnancy has not occurred, there is a tremendous drop-off of estrogen and progesterone in the blood. This results in increased secretion of FSH and LH. Hence, the whole cycle is repeated.

What Causes Menopause?

It is thought that menopause occurs when there are no eggs left in the ovaries. This "burning out" of the ovaries reflects the natural course of events. At birth, there are about 1 million eggs. By puberty this number has dropped to about 400,000. Only 400 or so of these ova will actually mature, during the reproductive years. By the time a woman reaches the age of 50, few eggs are left.

With menopause, the absence of active follicles results in a significant reduction in estrogen and progesterone levels. In response to this drop in estrogen, the pituitary increases secretion of FSH and LH. After menopause, FSH and LH are secreted continuously, in large quantities.

The postmenopausal woman no longer has any follicles to stimulate, so LH and FSH cause the ovaries as well as the adrenal glands to secrete increased amounts of male hormones (androgens), which can be converted to estrogens by the fat cells of the hips and thighs. Converted androgens account for most of the circulating estrogen in the postmenopausal woman, but the total amount of estrogen is still far below that of the woman in her reproductive years.

The Current View of Menopause: "Feminine" Forever?

In 1966, Robert A. Wilson, M.D., published a landmark book, *Feminine Forever*. In it Wilson presented the theory that menopause is an estrogen-deficiency disease that needs to be treated with estrogen to compensate for the normal decline of estrogen with aging.[1] According to Wilson, without estrogen replacement therapy, women are destined to become sexless "caricatures of their former selves . . . the equivalent of a eunuch."

Wilson's theory is now the dominant medical view of menopause. Is this view accurate? Or is menopause a natural life event? This book will help you decide the answers to these questions for yourself. Chapters 2 through 6 will discuss symptoms specific to menopause; Chapters 7 through 10 will discuss problems that are common in the postmenopausal years. You can decide the extent to which you think menopause is the culprit and whether these problems threaten your quality of life or identity as a woman. As in all matters relating to your health, you are the judge of what is barely noticeable, inconvenient, or intolerable.

Whatever you decide, if you are entering menopause, the current medical view of menopause places you in a dilemma. Should you remain, to use Wilson's terms, feminine forever? Or should you pass through this period of time naturally? If you are in this dilemma, you need to be aware of several facts. First, if you elect not to bear the risk of taking estrogen, natural methods can help alleviate the most bothersome menopausal symptoms as well as ensure long-term health. That being understood, the next factors to consider are the benefits and risks of estrogen replacement therapy.

Before assessing risks and benefits, however, consider the evolution of estrogen replacement therapy and what the future holds for it.

The Evolution of Estrogen Replacement Therapy

During the 1940s and 1950s, estrogen became a popular prescription for ameliorating the symptoms of menopause. By the time the 1970s arrived, estrogen replacement therapy was firmly entrenched as the medical treatment for menopause. Unfortunately, many women had to die of cancer of the lining of the uterus (endometrial cancer) before estrogen was identified as a major contributing factor.

It is now a well-established fact that estrogen replacement is associated with an increase in endometrial cancer. Extensive investigations resulted in this statistic: Women who take estrogen are 4 to 13 times more likely to develop endometrial cancer than women who are not taking estrogen.[2]

To weaken the link between estrogen and endometrial cancer, drug companies and physicians began recommending that estrogen be combined with progesterone. Estrogen replacement therapy thus became hormone replacement therapy (HRT). The combination of estrogen with progesterone (or, more accurately, a progestin) appears to have reduced the risk of endometrial cancer. However, HRT carries with it the stigma of increased risk of other cancers.[3] (This point will be discussed later in this chapter.) This stigma looms very large in the minds of many women and some physicians.

To deal with the issue of patient acceptance, drug companies are eagerly vying to develop estrogen and progesterone combinations that provide greater benefit than risk. Why? It is estimated that by the year 2015, 23% of the population in developed countries will be age 50 or older. The company that develops such a combination is virtually guaranteed a financial bonanza. Even in 1993, of all drug categories hormone replacement combinations for menopause ranked among the top in terms of dollar sales and number of prescriptions.

Why do so many doctors prescribe hormone replacement therapy? According to a recent review in a major medical journal, "the benefits of estrogen replacement therapy are undeniable." Yes, it is true. The benefits are undeniable, but what about the risks? Let's examine both of these in detail.

The Benefits of HRT

So what are the undeniable benefits of hormone replacement therapy? Relief of hot flashes and other menopausal symptoms, and a significant reduction in osteoporosis. Furthermore, although early studies linked estrogen use with an increased risk of cardiovascular disease, recent studies indicate that estrogen may offer some protection against heart disease and stroke.[4,5]

Before you get too excited about these beneficial effects of estrogen and HRT, remember that dietary, exercise, and lifestyle factors offer identical benefits without the risks. Furthermore, for menopausal symptoms, the use of short-term HRT (an HRT program of less than six months) provides only temporary relief; it is not a permanent cure, it just delays the inevitable. Long-term hormone replacement therapy is not justified for most women; the risks outweigh the benefits. The exceptions are women who have a high risk of developing osteoporosis.

One of the most publicized effects of estrogen is its role in maintaining bone health and preventing osteoporosis. The details of this role are provided in Chapter 7. In short, for women who are susceptible to osteoporosis and women who have already experienced significant bone loss, the benefits of hormonal therapy significantly outweigh its risks.

Does Your Osteoporosis Risk Warrant HRT?

To determine your risk of osteoporosis and the appropriateness of HRT for you, please take the self-test shown in Figure 1.1 (pages 9–11).

Before interpreting the results, reduce the risk factors that you have control over. Start an exercise program; quit smoking; do not drink alcohol, coffee, or soft drinks; take a high-quality calcium supplement. Just as important, consume a diet low in protein and high in vegetables. These changes could take as many as 150 points off your total score.

If, after reducing all the risk factors you can, your score on the osteoporosis risk test is still greater than 50, you are at significant risk for osteoporosis. Hormonal replacement therapy may be suitable for you, especially if you experienced an early menopause, had your ovaries surgically removed, or never had children.

Since both estrogen and progesterone have been shown to exert beneficial effects against bone loss and, in women with established bone loss, actually increase bone mass, estrogen-progesterone combinations are preferred to estrogen alone.[4,5] The exception is for women at high risk for breast cancer or women with a disease aggravated by estrogen. These diseases include breast cancer, active liver diseases, and certain cardiovascular diseases. In these cases, progesterone alone should be used.

SELF-TEST: Determining Your Risk of Osteoporosis

Choose the item in each category that best describes you, and fill in the point value for that item in the space to the right. You may choose more than one item in categories marked with an asterisk.

	Points	Score
Frame Size		
Small-boned or petite	10	
Medium frame, very lean	5	
Medium frame, average or heavy build	0	
Large frame, very lean	5	
Large frame, heavy build	0	*0*
Ethnic Background		
Caucasian	10	*10*
Asian	10	
Other	0	

Activity Level

How often do you walk briskly, jog, engage in aerobics/sports, or perform hard physical labor, of a duration of at least 30 continuous minutes?

Seldom	30	
1–2 times per week	20	*20*
3–4 times per week	5	
5 or more times per week	0	

Figure 1.1 The osteoporosis self-test

Figure 1.1 (continued)

	Points	Score
Smoking		
Smoke 10 or more cigarettes a day	20	_____
Smoke fewer than 10 cigarettes a day	10	_____
Quit smoking	5	_____
Never smoked	0	_O_
Personal Health Factors*		
Family history of osteoporosis	20	_____
Long-term corticosteroid use	20	_____
Long-term anticonvulsant use	20	_____
Drink more than 3 glasses of alcohol each week	20	_____
Drink more than 1 cup of coffee per day	10	_10_
Seldom get outside in the sunlight	10	_____
For women only:		
Had ovaries removed	10	_____
Premature menopause	10	_____
Had no children	10	_____
Dietary Factors*		
Consume more than 4 oz. of meat on a daily basis	20	_____
Drink soft drinks regularly	20	_____
Consume the equivalent of 3–5 servings of vegetables each day	-10	_____
Consume at least 1 cup of green leafy vegetables each day	-10	_____

*If applicable, choose more than one item in this category.

	Points	Score
Take a calcium supplement	−10	−10
Consume a vegetarian diet	−10	_____

Total score _____

The Risks of HRT

Of all the risks of HRT, the risk of cancer is of most concern.

HRT and Cancer

Researchers have conducted over 30 studies to establish or quantify the effect of HRT on cancer risk.[6-9] Unfortunately, despite intense investigation, these studies have not provided any clear-cut answers. The bottom line is that nobody really knows for sure what impact HRT has on cancer, but there is enough evidence to warrant concern.

The form of cancer most likely to be adversely affected by HRT is breast cancer. Breast cancer is already the most common cancer in women. Current estimates are that one in nine women in the United States will develop breast cancer. Since estrogens play a critical role in the development of most breast cancers, it only makes sense that additional estrogens may promote breast cancer.

When all the studies of the HRT–breast cancer link are examined collectively, experts calculate that HRT is associated with a 1% to 30% increase in the risk of breast cancer.[7-9] Most of the studies that showed a positive correlation were conducted in Europe. In comparison, only a few U.S. studies have shown hormone replacement therapy as a factor that increases the risk of breast cancer. These results raise some interesting questions. Are American researchers biased? Is the failure to show an increased risk for breast cancer in American women due to the fact that American women are already at high risk for breast cancer? And why are American researchers so defensive about the positive findings in the European studies?

The answers to these questions may reflect the fact that the U.S. medical establishment has enthusiastically been recommending estrogen and HRT for many years. No researcher or physician wants to admit that a drug that they have so enthusiastically recommended is now linked to a dreaded disease like cancer.

Based on the current evidence, and until the issue of whether HRT increases the risk of breast cancer is resolved, I believe that well-intentioned physicians and their female patients are better off avoiding hormone replacement therapy.

Other Side Effects of HRT

The side effects of estrogen and progesterone are listed in the *Physicians' Desk Reference* and on inserts in packages of products containing these hormones. The long lists are frightening. In addition to the risk of cancer, estrogen and progesterone increase the risk of developing blood clots, which could lead to a stroke or heart attack, and gallstones. Estrogen and progesterone should absolutely not be used during the first four months of pregnancy.

Other side effects of estrogen and progesterone include:

Nausea

Breast tenderness

Symptoms similar to those of premenstrual tension syndrome (PMS)

Depression

Liver disorders

Enlargement of uterine fibroids

Fluid retention

Blood sugar disturbances

Headaches

Note, however, that the preceding side effects are most often linked to taking the estrogen and progesterone contained in birth control pills. Since the doses of estrogen and progesterone used for menopause are much lower than those for oral contraception, these side effects are usually not as common when used for menopause.

Types of HRT

Suppose you have weighed all the evidence and chosen HRT for long-term therapy (because of very high risk of osteoporosis) or short-term relief. Your next step—and it is very important—is to participate in choosing the dosage pattern and type of product that will best meet your needs.

Dosage Components and Patterns

Experts do not agree on a "best" program of HRT. Programs differ in terms of the hormones administered and how often they are administered. The two primary programs are unopposed estrogen therapy and combined estrogen therapy.

Unopposed Estrogen Therapy   When estrogen is given alone, without a progestin, it is known as unopposed estrogen therapy. This regime carries with it a high risk of endometrial cancer and possibly other cancers, including breast cancer. Unopposed estrogen can be given either "continuously" (every day) or during 25-day cycles separated by three to six days without estrogen.

Combined Estrogen Therapy   In an effort to reduce the risk of endometrial cancer, estrogen is often given in combination with a progestin, such as progesterone. The hormones can be given either in a cyclical fashion or continuously. The cyclical fashion involves taking estrogen for 25 days and progestin for the last 10 to 12 days of the cycle.

Three- to six-day hormone-free intervals follow, during which planned bleeding occurs. In other words, with cyclical administration, periods continue in about 90% of women.

To prevent monthly bleeding, estrogen and progesterone can be given each day, without a hormone-free interval. This regime is known as combined continuous hormone replacement therapy. When administered according to recommended guidelines (the lowest dose of estrogen possible along with 2.5 milligrams of medroxyprogesterone acetate), combined continuous HRT offers several advantages over other popular regimes. The advantages include:

- Avoidance of cyclical bleeding
- Continuous protection of the endometrium against the cancer-causing effects of estrogen
- Lower requirements for daily and cumulative amounts of progestins
- Avoidance of symptoms of PMS, which often accompany estrogen use
- Prolongation of the synergistic effects of estrogen and progesterone on bone integrity
- Regression of uterine fibroids
- Prevention of rare conceptions by promotion of endometrial atrophy (shrinkage)
- Convenient administration, which leads to patient compliance

Based on current evidence, I believe that combined continuous HRT is the best HRT program in terms of benefits outweighing risks.[4,5]

Hormone Products

As for the best type of estrogen to use, "natural" estrogens are preferred to synthetic versions. Examples of

natural estrogens commonly used in hormone replacem
therapy include:

Conjugated estrogens (Premarin, Genisis)
Esterified estrogens (Evex, Menest)
Micronized 17-beta-estradiol (Estrace)
Transdermal 17-beta-estradiol (Estraderm, Systen)

The most commonly used forms are the conjugated estrogens, such as Premarin. Conjugated estrogens are broken
down in the body to form active estrogens, such as 17-beta-
estradiol. Unfortunately, the liver metabolizes many of the
active estrogens before they have the opportunity to produce
effects. What is more, the most active estrogen, 17-beta-
estradiol, is not absorbed well orally. Therefore, the patient
must take relatively large oral doses of conjugated estrogens.

The active estrogen 17-beta-estradiol is absorbed very
well through the skin, however. This form of estrogen is used
in the newer estrogen patches as well as vaginal creams.

Estrogen patches are preferable to oral conjugated
estrogens for several reasons, but primarily because the
delivery system approximates the female body's own natural
estrogen secretions. The patches deliver 17-beta-estradiol
into the bloodstream in a slow, sustained manner. Estrogen-
containing patches appear to be safer, in all respects, than
oral estrogens. The patches are applied to the skin and
changed twice per week.

What is the best form of progesterone? The "natural"
derivative of progesterone, medroxyprogesterone acetate,
is preferred to synthetic versions such as megestrol, nor-
ethindrone, and norgestrel. Examples of medoxyproges-
terone products are Provera, Cycrin, and Amen.

Menopause as a Social Construct

The biomechanical model of health that most physicians
adhere to leaves little room for other explanatory models.

In the case of menopause, the biomechanical model focuses on the physiological process due to ovarian decline. But what about the psychological and cultural aspects of menopause?

There is undeniably a physiological process involved in menopause; however, menopause is much more than a biological event. Social and cultural factors contribute greatly to how women react to menopause.[10] In our current society, menopause is viewed as a deficiency disease.

Modern society has placed great value on the allure of everlasting youth. Our culture tends to devalue older women. This devaluation is deeply entrenched in our mental programming. You can find examples of it in our children's books, fairy tales, television, and movies. Advocates of a social and cultural explanation of menopause often point to this cultural devaluing of older women as the root of the negativity associated with achieving menopause.

In many cultures of the world, women look forward to menopause because it actually brings with it greater respect. Achieving an advanced age is viewed as a sign of divine blessing and great wisdom. The cultural view of menopause relates directly to menopause symptoms.[11] If the cultural view of menopause is largely negative, as in the United States, symptoms are quite common. In contrast, if menopause is associated with little negativity or viewed in a positive light, symptoms are far less frequent.

Studies of menopausal women in many traditional cultures demonstrate that most will pass through menopause without hot flashes, vaginitis, and other symptoms common to menopausal women in developed countries. In addition, osteoporosis is extremely rare, despite the fact that the average woman in many traditional societies lives at least 30 years after menopause.

The question is obvious: Do women in traditional cultures experience the same hormonal changes that women in industrialized nations experience? Surprisingly, the answer is *yes*. The next question: If women in traditional cultures experience the same hormonal changes, why don't they experience the symptoms of menopause? The answer: These women have an entirely different view of menopause.

One of the most detailed studies of the effects of culture on menopause involved rural Mayan Indians.[11] Detailed medical histories and examinations (which included physical exams, hormone concentrations, and bone density studies) were performed on 52 postmenopausal women. According to the data, no woman experienced hot flashes or any other menopausal symptom and not one single woman showed evidence of osteoporosis. These results occurred despite the fact that the hormonal patterns of the Mayan women were identical to those of postmenopausal women living in the United States.

The researchers in this study felt that the attitude the Mayan women had toward menopause was responsible for the difference in their symptomless passage through menopause. The Mayan women saw menopause as a positive event that would provide them acceptance as respected elders as well as relief from childbearing. This attitude is much different than the dominant attitude toward menopause common in industrialized societies.

The lifestyle of women in the United States differs greatly from that of the Mayan women in the study. The two groups eat different foods, have different levels of physical activity, and live in different climates. All the factors could contribute toward the way each group experiences menopause. This study raises an interesting question, however. If our society adopted a different view of menopause, to what extent might the experience of menopause change? Since the social attitude is unlikely to change in the very near future, I strongly encourage readers to become aware of how they view themselves and older women. Do not buy into our youth-oriented prejudices and distortion. Value yourself and those who have attained the divine blessing and wisdom that comes with menopause.

The Doctor-Patient Relationship

Is estrogen replacement therapy necessary? For the majority of women, the answer is a resounding no. Does this mean you should not follow your doctor's advice if he or she has prescribed estrogen? Not necessarily. Communicate with your physician about your health goals. I encourage you to find a doctor with whom you can develop an effective and trusting relationship. To find a naturopathic doctor (N.D.) or holistic medical doctor in your area, call or write:

> The American Association of Naturopathic Physicians
> P.O. Box 20386
> Seattle, WA 98102
> (206) 323-7610

or

> The American Holistic Medical Association
> 4101 Lake Boone Trail, #201
> Raleigh, NC 26707
> (919) 787-5146

Although this book is largely designed to help you take control of your own health, you must be evaluated and monitored by a physician—especially if you are menopausal. If you are experiencing the symptoms of menopause, I recommend that you see your primary care physician or gynecologist for a baseline evaluation. This evaluation includes:

> Detailed personal and family medical history
> Breast exam and instructions on self-examination of breasts
> Pelvic examination

The following laboratory tests:

    Complete blood count

    Blood-chemistry panel

    Cholesterol evaluation, including HDL, LDL, and VLDL

    Thyroid function panel, including T_3, T_4, and TSH

Baseline mammography (if indicated)

Baseline bone densitometry

After this initial evaluation, repeat these tests every year. The bone-density studies can be used as a gauge to determine whether hormone replacement therapy is necessary.

II

The Natural Approach to Menopause Symptoms

The foremost goal in the natural approach to menopause is to provide relief from common symptoms. This section will focus on the most common complaints of menopause: hot flashes, headaches, thinning of the lining of the vagina (atrophic vaginitis), frequent urinary tract infections, cold hands and feet, forgetfulness, the inability to concentrate, and depression.

Rather than use estrogens to counteract these symptoms artificially, the natural approach focuses on improving physiology. This improvement can be accomplished through diet, exercise, nutritional supplementation, and the use of plant-based medicines.

2

Hot Flashes

H ot flashes are the most common symptoms of menopause. A hot flash is a rise in skin temperature and a flushing of the skin (peripheral vasodilation). In the typical hot flash, the skin, especially of the head and neck, becomes red and warm for a few seconds to 2 minutes; chills follow. Hot flashes can be accompanied by other symptoms, including increased heart rate, headaches, dizziness, weight gain, fatigue, and insomnia.

In the United States, about 65% to 75% of menopausal women experience hot flashes to some degree. Hot flashes are often the very first sign that menopause is approaching—they may begin prior to the cessation of menses. In most cases, hot flashes are most uncomfortable in the first to second years after menopause. As the body adapts to decreased estrogen levels, hot flashes typically subside.

..ole of the Hypothalamus and Endorphins

Many of the symptoms of menopause, especially hot flashes, appear to be a result of altered function of the hypothalamus. The hypothalamus is the part of the brain that is at the center of the head, just above the pituitary gland. It serves as the bridge between the nervous system and the hormonal (endocrine) system. The hypothalamus is responsible for the control of many body functions, including body temperature, metabolic rate, sleep patterns, reactions to stress, libido, mood, and the release of pituitary hormones. Critical to proper functioning of the hypothalamus are compounds known as endorphins.

Endorphins are also called endogenous opioids, or endogenous morphine. These names highlight the similarity between endorphins and opium or morphine. These natural opioids are the body's own pain-relieving and antidepressant compounds. They act as chemical messengers within the brain and endocrine system. Endorphins are the vehicles that allow the hypothalamus to perform its vital functions.

Several natural measures are thought to promote endorphin output. Most notable are exercise and acupuncture. The endorphin-releasing effects of exercise and acupuncture imply that they might be effective in relieving many menopausal symptoms, especially hot flashes.

The Natural Approach to Hot Flashes

Natural measures that address some of the underlying reasons for hot flashes include exercise, diet, nutritional supplementation, and plant-based medicines.

Exercise and Hot Flashes

One hypothesis suggested that impaired endorphin activity within the hypothalamus is a major factor in provoking hot flashes. This hypothesis led researchers in Sweden to design a study to determine the effect of regular physical exercise on the frequency of hot flashes.[1] In the study, the frequency of moderate and severe hot flashes was investigated in 79 postmenopausal women who took part in physical exercise on a regular basis. The data from this group was compared to data from a control group of 866 postmenopausal women between 52 and 54 years old. Both groups filled out detailed questionnaires that included the grading of hot flashes as mild, moderate, and severe. The women in the regular exercise group also answered questions about their physical activity.

The results of the study clearly demonstrated that regular physical exercise definitely lowered the frequency and severity of hot flashes. Several interesting points arise from the results: (1) The women in the exercising group passed through a natural menopause, without the use of hormone replacement therapy, and (2) the physically active women who had no hot flashes whatsoever spent an average of only 3.5 hours per week exercising; women who exercised less than this amount were more likely to have hot flashes.

The benefits of regular exercise on mood and the health of bone and the cardiovascular system are well known. Add to these benefits the positive results about reduction of the frequency and severity of hot flashes, and the message is obvious. Regular physical exercise is a critical prescription for health. Chapter 13 will provide the guidelines necessary for constructing an effective exercise routine.

Dietary Recommendations to Minimize Hot Flashes

Although no specific dietary therapy has been investigated for the treatment of hot flashes, dietary therapy has been studied in the treatment of atrophic vaginitis (see Chapter 3). To provide dietary support for yourself during menopause, follow the dietary guidelines in Chapters 3 and 11. Some specific foods to eat for hot flashes include fennel, celery, and parsley; soy; high-lignan flaxseed oil; and nuts and seeds.

Fennel, celery, and parsley are members of the *Umbelliferae* group of plants. Members of this group, called umbellifers, typically contain active estrogenlike substances known as phytoestrogens. Fennel is particularly rich in phytoestrogens and possesses confirmed estrogenic action.[2] Other foods rich in phytoestrogens include soy, nuts, whole grains, apples, and alfalfa. The high intake of phytoestrogens is thought to explain why hot flashes and other menopausal symptoms rarely occur in cultures consuming a predominantly plant-based diet.[3]

The beneficial effects of soy will be discussed throughout this book. Most notable are its effects in atrophic vaginitis and the prevention of breast cancer. Regular consumption of soy foods may help lessen hot flashes as well.

The beneficial effects of lignans on estrogen metabolism will be discussed in Chapter 8. These effects may also prove to be of benefit in treating hot flashes. Use a high-lignan flaxseed oil as a salad dressing. Just 1 to 2 tablespoons per day is all that is required.

Nuts and seeds are also good sources of compounds known as phytosterols. These plant compounds are structurally similar to estrogen and other steroid hormones. Chemists think that the body may be able to utilize phytosterols as if they were estrogen. Try and consume at least ½ cup of raw nuts (not peanuts or macadamia) or seeds each day.

Nutritional Supplements That Minimize Hot Flashes

In general, the dietary guidelines provided in Chapter 11 are quite appropriate in the treatment of hot flashes. Clinical studies have shown, however, that several nutrients are particularly effective in relieving hot flashes. These nutrients are vitamin E, hesperidin in combination with vitamin C, and gamma-oryzanol.

Vitamin E　In the late 1940s, several clinical studies demonstrated that vitamin E relieved hot flashes and menopausal vaginal complaints.[4-6] Unfortunately, there have been no further clinical investigations. It is often recommended that vitamin E be taken at a daily dose of 800 IU (international units). After the hot flashes have subsided, the dosage can be reduced to 400 IU.

Hesperidin and Vitamin C　Hesperidin is a flavonoid found in citrus fruit. Like many other flavonoids, hesperidin improves vascular integrity and relieves capillary permeability. Combined with vitamin C, hesperidin and other citrus flavonoids can provide relief from hot flashes.

In one clinical study, 94 women suffering from hot flashes were given a formula containing 900 milligrams of hesperidin, 300 milligrams of hesperidin methyl chalcone (another citrus flavonoid), and 1,200 milligrams of vitamin C daily.[7] At the end of one month, symptoms were relieved in 53% of the patients and reduced in 34%. In addition to hot flashes, improvements were noted in nocturnal leg cramps, nosebleeds, and easy bruising. The only side effect noted was a slightly offensive odor and a tendency for perspiration to discolor the patient's clothing.

Hesperidin and citrus flavonoid products are available at health food stores. To use these products and vitamin C to treat hot flashes, use the dosages cited in the preceding paragraph.

Gamma-Oryzanol　Gamma-oryzanol (ferulic acid) is a growth-promoting substance found in grains and isolated from rice bran oil. In the treatment of hot flashes, its primary action is to enhance pituitary function and promote endorphin release by the hypothalamus. Gamma-oryzanol was first shown to be effective in treating menopausal symptoms, including hot flashes, in the early 1960s.[8] Subsequent studies have further documented its effectiveness.[9]

In one of the earlier studies, eight menopausal women and 13 women whose ovaries had been surgically removed were given 300 milligrams of gamma-oryzanol daily. At the end of the 38-day trial, over 67% of the women had a 50% or greater reduction in their menopausal symptoms.[8] In a more recent study, a daily 300-milligram dose of gamma-oryzanol was even more effective: Of the women studied, 85% reported improvement in their symptoms.[9]

Gamma-oryzanol is an extremely safe natural substance. No significant side effects have ever been produced in experiments or clinical studies. In addition to improving the symptoms of menopause, gamma-oryzanol has also lowered blood cholesterol and triglyceride levels.[10]

Plant-Based Medicines That Minimize Hot Flashes

Many plant-based medicines have been shown to exhibit a beneficial effect on the female glandular system. This effect is thought to be a result of phytoestrogens in the plants as well as the ability of plant compounds to improve blood flow to the female organs. The plant-based medicines nourish and tone the female glandular and organ system rather than exert a druglike effect. This nonspecific mode of action makes many plants useful in the treatment of a broad range of women's conditions.

Phytoestrogens are components of many medicinal plants. Historically, these plants were used to treat conditions that are now treated by estrogens. Phytoestrogen-containing plants offer significant advantages over estrogens in the treatment of menopausal symptoms. Both synthetic and natural estrogens may pose significant health risks, including an increased risk of cancer, gallbladder disease, and thromboembolic disease (stroke, heart attack, and the like).

Phytoestrogens, in contrast, have not been associated with these side effects. In fact, experimental studies of animals have demonstrated that phytoestrogens are extremely effective in inhibiting mammary tumors not only because they occupy estrogen receptors, but because they activate other anticancer mechanisms.[3,11,12]

Phytoestrogens in plants are capable of exerting estrogenic effects. At the most, however, the activity of phytoestrogens is only 2% as strong as that of estrogen.[13,14] However, because of this low activity, phytoestrogens have a balancing action on estrogen effects. Because phytoestrogens have some estrogenic activity, they cause an increase in estrogen effect if estrogen levels are low. Since phytoestrogens bind to estrogen-receptor binding sites, they compete with estrogen. Therefore, if estrogen levels are high, estrogen effects decrease.

Because of this balancing action of phytoestrogens, it is common to find the same plant recommended for conditions of estrogen excess (such as premenstrual syndrome) as well as conditions of estrogen deficiency (such as menopause and menstrual abnormalities). Many of these plants have been termed uterine tonics.

The four most useful herbs in the treatment of hot flashes are angelica, or dong quai (*Angelica sinensis*); licorice root (*Glycyrrhiza glabra*), chasteberry (*Vitex agnus-castus*), and black cohosh (*Cimicifuga racemosa*). These herbs have been used for centuries to lessen a variety of female complaints.

Although these herbs may be effective individually, combining them may produce even greater benefit. Most major suppliers of herbal products feature formulas containing these herbs. Use well-respected brands and follow the dosage instructions on the label. Brief discussions of these important plants follow.

Angelica   In Asia, angelica is called dong quai, and its reputation for healing is perhaps second only to that of ginseng. Predominantly regarded as a "female" remedy, angelica has been used to treat menopausal symptoms (especially hot flashes), as well as dysmenorrhea (painful menstruation), amenorrhea (absence of menstruation), metrorrhagia (abnormal menstruation), and to promote a healthy pregnancy and easy delivery.

Angelica causes an initial increase in uterine contraction followed by relaxation.[15] In addition, administration of angelica to mice resulted in an increase of uterine weight and an increase in glucose utilization by the liver and uterus.[16] These effects reflect estrogenic activities.

The effectiveness of angelica in treating hot flashes may be due to a combination of mild estrogenic effects and those of components that help stabilize blood vessels.[17]

Dosage (take these amounts, three times daily)

Powdered root or as tea	1 to 2 grams (1 to 2 teaspoons per 8 ounces of hot water)
Tincture (1:5)	4 milliliters (1 teaspoon)
Fluid extract	1 milliliter (¼ teaspoon)

Licorice Root   The medicinal use of licorice in both Western and Eastern cultures dates back several thousand years. In addition to being used for a variety of female disorders, licorice root was used primarily as an expectorant and antitussive in the treatment of respiratory tract infections and asthma. Traditionally, it was also used to treat peptic ulcers, malaria, abdominal pain, insomnia, and infection. Its effectiveness for many of these uses has been substantiated by modern research.

Licorice is particularly useful in treating premenstrual syndrome, or PMS. PMS has been attributed to an increase in the estrogen-progesterone ratio. Licorice is believed to reduce estrogen while increasing progesterone.

In regard to menopause, it is thought that the estrogenlike activity of licorice is responsible for many of its beneficial effects, but its effects on progesterone may also be important.[18,19]

Dosage (take these amounts, three times daily)

Powdered root or as tea	1 to 2 grams (1 to 2 teaspoons per 8 ounces of hot water)
Fluid extract (1:1)	4 milliliters (1 teaspoon)
Solid (dry powdered) extract (4:1)	250 to 500 milligrams

Chasteberries The chaste tree is native to the Mediterranean area. Its berries have long been used for female complaints. As its name signifies, chasteberries were used to suppress libido. Scientific investigation has shown that the chemical components of chasteberry have profound effects on pituitary function.[20] It is possible that its beneficial effects in treating menopause are due to its role in altering LH and FSH secretion.

Dosage (take these amounts, three times daily)

Powdered berries or as tea	1 to 2 grams (1 to 2 teaspoons per 8 ounces of hot water)
Fluid extract (1:1)	4 milliliters (1 teaspoon)
Solid (dry powdered) extract (4:1)	250 to 500 milligrams

Black Cohosh Black cohosh was widely used by the American Indians and later by American colonists for the relief of menstrual cramps and menopause. Recent scientific investigation has upheld the effectiveness of black cohosh as a treatment for dysmenorrhea and menopause. Clinical studies have shown extracts of black cohosh to relieve not only hot flashes, but also depression and vaginal atrophy.[21]

In addition to exerting vascular effects, black cohosh reduces LH levels; thus, the plant has a significant estrogenic effect.

Dosage (take these amounts, three times daily)

Powdered berries or as tea	1 to 2 grams (1 to 2 teaspoons per 8 ounces of hot water)
Fluid extract (1:1)	4 milliliters (1 teaspoon)
Solid (dry powdered) extract (4:1)	250 to 500 milligrams

Final Comments

As this chapter makes evident, natural measures can help alleviate hot flashes. Here are some concise recommendations:

1. Develop a regular exercise program.
2. Follow the dietary guidelines presented in Chapter 11.
3. Follow the guidelines for nutritional supplementation, given in Chapter 12.
4. Use one of the plant-based medicines discussed in this chapter at an appropriate dosage. Or, use a combination formula that features compounds from several of these plants. Most suppliers of herbal products offer such combination formulas. For example, in my clinical practice, I recommend a formula containing extracts of angelica, licorice root, chasteberry, and black cohosh plus vitamin C, hesperidin, and extracts of false unicorn root and fennel.
5. If additional support is needed, try taking 300 milligrams of gamma-oryzanol each day.

3

Atrophic Vaginitis

After menopause, the vaginal lining may become thin and dry because of the lack of estrogen. During the reproductive years, estrogen stimulates the cells that line the vagina; the estrogen helps maintain proper moisture and cell structure. Without the effects of estrogen, menopausal and postmenopausal women may experience painful intercourse, an increased susceptibility to infection, and vaginal itching or burning. The medical term used to describe this condition is *atrophic vaginitis*.

The Natural Approach to Atrophic Vaginitis

To treat atrophic vaginitis, follow the guidelines provided in Chapter 2, in regard to the treatment of hot flashes. To provide immediate relief, one of the most popular natural measures is the topical use of vitamin E oil, creams, ointments, or suppositories. Vitamin E is usually quite effective in relieving the dryness and irritation of atrophic vaginitis as well as other forms of vaginitis.[1]

Taking vitamin E internally may also be of benefit. In a study conducted in 1942, vitamin E supplements, when taken for at least four weeks, not only improved symptoms, but also improved the blood supply to the vaginal wall.[2] A follow-up study published in 1949 demonstrated that high-dose vitamin E (400 IU [international units] daily) was effective in about 50% of postmenopausal women with atrophic vaginitis.[3]

An especially important dietary treatment is to increase the consumption of soy foods. As briefly mentioned in Chapter 2, soy contains phytoestrogens. Specifically, the isoflavones and phytosterols of soybeans produce a mild estrogenic effect. One cup of soybeans provides approximately 300 milligrams of isoflavones. This level would be the equivalent of about 0.45 milligrams of conjugated estrogens or one tablet of Premarin.[4] However, while estrogen replacement therapy may increase the risk of cancer, the consumption of soy foods is associated with a significant reduction in cancer risk.[4,5]

One study of postmenopausal women compared a group that consumed soy foods (enough to provide about 200 milligrams of isoflavone) to a control group that did not eat soy foods.[4] For the women who ate soy foods, the number of superficial cells in the lining of the vagina increased. This increase offset vaginal drying and irritation.

Soy and Soy Foods

The soybean plant (*Glycine max*) is native to China, where it has been cultivated for food for well over 13,000 years. The ancient Chinese considered the soybean their most important crop and a necessity for life. Thanks largely to the United States, where over 50% of the world's soybeans are produced, the soybean plant is now the most widely grown and utilized legume. It accounts for well over 50% of global legume production. In terms of dollar value, the soybean is the most important crop in the United States; it ranks above corn, wheat, and cotton. Unfortunately, in the United States, soybeans are still used primarily for animal feed (protein meal) and for its oils. However, since the 1970s, there has been a marked increase in both the consumption of traditional soy foods—such as tofu, tempeh, and miso—and in the development of so-called second-generation soy foods, which simulate traditional meat and dairy products.

The increase in soy food consumption is attributed to a number of factors, including economics, health benefits, and environmental concerns. In terms of cost, soy beans provide a great amount of nutrition per acre. In fact, an acre of soybeans can provide nearly 20 times the protein produced by an acre used for raising beef cattle. The use and reliance on soy will grow as the world's population continues to grow and its food supply continues to shrink.

Practical Guidelines for Increasing Soy Intake

Soybeans can be utilized in cooked or sprouted form, either on their own or in recipes. Soybeans can substitute for other beans in soups, stews, casseroles, and other dishes. In addition, there are many other soy foods and soy food ingredients.

Soy Alternatives The typical health food store and some supermarkets offer soy alternatives to many animal-based foods, including hamburgers, hot dogs, sausage, frozen desserts, and cheese. Some of these soy alternatives are actually quite delicious. Modern food technology is being put to good use to make healthful versions of common American foods.

Soy Flour Excluding soybeans used for oil, more than 90% of the soybeans consumed in the United States are in the form of soy protein products. These products include soy flour, soy protein concentrates, and soy protein isolates. Such products are made from defatted soybean flakes, and their protein content ranges from 40% to 90%. The lower the protein content, the higher the level of isoflavonoids. Therefore, in dealing with the symptoms of menopause, low-protein products, such as soy flour, are superior to high-protein isolates. Soy flour can be used to create baked goods—breads, rolls, buns, bagels, pancakes, waffles, and so on. Soy flour not only greatly improves protein quality, but also provides some isoflavonoids.

Soy Milk   Soy milk is increasing in popularity because of improvements in commercial production. The traditional way to produce soy milk is to soak the beans in water, grind the soaked beans, and filter the resulting mass. Commercially available soy milks may be produced in this manner or produced from soy protein concentrates (70% protein) and isolates (90% protein). The important thing to remember is that products made from whole soybeans are higher in isoflavonoid content than those produced from soy protein concentrates.

On its own, soy milk is not that palatable. To enhance the flavor, a variety of natural flavors—such as vanilla, chocolate, and carob—are used. There are even soy milk frozen desserts that offer a delicious and healthy alternative to ice cream.

Tofu   Tofu, or bean curd, is now a well-known food. After soy sauce, it is the biggest seller among soy foods in the United States. Tofu is made by adding calcium or magnesium salts (nigari) to soy milk. The salts coagulate the proteins. The liquid (whey) is discarded and the curds are pressed to form a cohesive bond. The degree of pressing determines whether the product is soft, regular, or firm tofu.

From a nutritional perspective, tofu is an excellent food. Substituting tofu for cheese, for example, has lowered blood cholesterol levels, both in men and women. Although tofu is rather bland on its own, it readily takes on the flavor of the ingredients it is cooked with. This makes it extremely versatile. Tofu serves as the major component of many second-generation soy products.

Final Recommendations

Women with atrophic vaginitis should try to avoid substances that dry the membranes of the body, including antihistamines, alcohol, caffeine, and diuretics. In addition, it is critical that the body stay well hydrated. Drink at least 2 quarts of liquid, preferably pure water or fresh juice, each day.

Wear clothes made from natural fibers, particularly cotton. Natural fibers allow the skin to breathe.

Regular intercourse is beneficial; it increases blood flow to vaginal tissues, which helps improve tone and lubrication. However, when having intercourse, be sure to use an effective lubricant, such as K-Y Jelly.

4

Bladder Infections

About 15% of menopausal women experience frequent bladder infections. The typical symptoms of a bladder infection can include a burning pain during urination; increased urinary frequency; nighttime urination; a turbid, foul-smelling, or dark urine; and lower abdominal pain.

Most bladder infections are caused by bacteria; however, clinical symptoms and the presence of significant amounts of bacteria in the urine (as evidenced by culturing) do not always correlate. Only 60% of women with the typical symptoms of urinary tract infection actually have significant levels of bacteria in their urine.

In general, the diagnosis of a bladder infection is made on the basis of signs, symptoms, and urinary findings. Microscopic examination of the infected urine will reveal high levels of white blood cells and bacteria. Culturing the urine may determine the quantity and type of bacteria involved. *Escherichia coli*, or *E. coli*, bacteria is responsible for about 90% of bladder infections.

Urine, as it is secreted by the kidneys, is sterile until it reaches the urethra. The urethra is the tube that transports the urine from the bladder to the urethral opening. Bacteria are introduced into the urethra from vaginal secretions.

The body has many defenses against bacterial growth in the urinary tract. Urine flow tends to wash away bacteria. The surface of the bladder has antimicrobial properties. The pH of the urine inhibits the growth of many bacteria, and the body quickly secretes white blood cells to control the bacteria.

Chronic Interstitial Cystitis

Cystitis is a word for inflammation of the urinary bladder. Chronic interstitial cystitis is a persistent form of cystitis not due to infection. Food allergies have been shown to produce cystitis in some patients.[1-3] Repeated ingestion of a food allergen could explain the chronic nature of interstitial cystitis.

The best way to determine whether a food allergy is a factor is to use the elimination and challenge method. In other words, a person is placed on a limited diet; commonly eaten foods are eliminated and replaced with either hypoallergenic foods or foods the patient rarely eats. The fewer the allergic foods, the greater the ease of establishing a diagnosis with an elimination diet. The standard elimination diet consists of lamb, chicken, potatoes, rice, banana, apple, and a cabbage-family vegetable (cabbage, Brussels sprouts, or broccoli, for example). Variations of the elimination diet are suitable in cases where one of the foods in the standard diet is suspected of causing a problem. The important point is that the person eat no suspected allergens.

The individual stays on this limited diet for at least one week and up to one month. If the symptoms are related to food sensitivity, they will typically disappear by the fifth or sixth day of the diet. If the symptoms do not disappear, it is possible that a reaction to a food in the elimination diet is responsible. In such a case, an even more restricted diet must be utilized.

After one week, individual foods are reintroduced according to a plan. Methods range from reintroducing a single food every two days to reintroducing a food at every meal. Usually, after the "cleansing" period, the patient has developed an increased sensitivity to offending foods.

Reintroduction of an allergen typically produces a more severe or recognizable symptom than before. The patient must keep a careful, detailed record of when foods were reintroduced and what symptoms appeared upon reintroduction. In addition, tracking the wrist pulse during reintroduction can be helpful because pulse changes may occur when the patient eats an allergen. Hopefully, when the allergen is eliminated, chronic interstitial cystitis will disappear.

The Natural Approach to Bladder Infections

The primary goal in the natural approach to treating bladder infections is enhancing normal host-protective measures against urinary tract infection. Specifically, this means enhancing the flow of urine through proper hydration, promoting a pH to inhibit the growth of the infecting organism, and preventing bacterial adherence to the endothelial cells of the bladder. In addition, several botanical medicines can be employed.

Increase Urine Flow

Increasing urine flow can be easily achieved by increasing the amount of liquids consumed. Ideally, the liquids consumed should be in the form of pure water, fresh juices diluted with an equal amount of water, and herbal teas. The patient should be encouraged to drink at least 64 ounces of liquids from this group, with at least half of this amount being water. The patient should avoid soft drinks, concentrated fruit drinks, coffee, and alcoholic beverages.

In the treatment of urinary tract infections, cranberries and cranberry juice have been shown to be quite effective.[4-6] In one study, 16 ounces of cranberry juice per day produced beneficial effects in 73% of the subjects (44 females and 16 males), who had active urinary tract infections.[4] Furthermore, withdrawal of the cranberry juice resulted in recurrence of bladder infection in 61%.

Many people believe that the action of cranberry juice is due to acidification of the urine and the antibacterial effects of a cranberry component, hippuric acid. These are probably not the major mechanisms of action.[7,8] To acidify the urine, a person would have to drink at least 1 quart of cranberry juice at one sitting. In addition, the concentration of hippuric acid in the urine as a result of drinking cranberry juice is not sufficient to inhibit bacteria. In the treatment of bladder infection, positive effects from drinking cranberry juice have been noted in cases in which the patients drank only 16 ounces of cranberry juice per day. This indicates that a mechanism other than acidification and antibacterial effects is at work.

Recent studies have shown that components in cranberry juice reduce the ability of *E. coli* to adhere to the lining of the bladder and urethra.[9,10] For bacteria to infect, they must first adhere to the mucosa. By interfering with adherence, cranberry juice greatly reduces the likelihood of infection and helps the body fight off infection. This is the most likely explanation for the positive effects of cranberry juice on bladder infections.

One study of seven juices (cranberry, blueberry, grapefruit, guava, mango, orange, and pineapple) showed that, of the seven, only cranberry and blueberry juices contain this inhibitor.[10] Blueberry juice is a suitable alternative to cranberry juice in the treatment of bladder infections.

Most cranberry juices on the market contain one-third cranberry juice mixed with water and sugar. Sugar has a detrimental effect on the immune system.[11,12] Therefore, use of sweetened cranberry juice cannot be recommended. Fresh cranberry juice (sweetened with apple or grape juice) or blueberry juice is preferred. Cranberry extracts in pill form are commercially available. The amount of cranberry extract taken daily should be the equivalent of 16 ounces of cranberry juice. There is no known toxicity as a result of cranberry ingestion.

Acidify or Alkalinize the Urine?

Although many physicians and women believe acidifying the urine is the best approach in addressing cystitis, several arguments can be made for alkalinizing the urine. First of all, it is often very difficult to acidify the urine. Many popular methods of acidification, such as taking ascorbic acid supplements and drinking cranberry juice, have very little effect on pH at commonly prescribed doses.

The best argument for alkalinizing the urine is that it appears to be more effective, especially for women without evidence of bacteria in their urine. The best method for alkalinizing the urine seems to be the use of citrate salts—potassium citrate and sodium citrate, for example. These salts are rapidly absorbed and metabolized, without affecting gastric pH or producing a laxative effect. They are excreted partly as carbonate, thus raising the pH of the urine.

Potassium citrate and sodium citrate have long been employed in the treatment of lower urinary tract infections. They are often used as a stopgap treatment while the physician is waiting for the results of a urine culture. Several clinical studies support this practice. For example, in one study, women with symptoms of a urinary tract infection were given a 4-gram dose of sodium citrate every 8 hours for 48 hours.[13] Of the 64 women evaluated, 80% of the women experienced relief of symptoms, 12% experienced deterioration of symptoms, and 91.8% rated the treatment as acceptable. Of the 64 women, 19 had positive bacterial cultures. In the group of women with proven bacterial infection, 7 of the 10 women with urethral pain and 13 of the 18 women with painful or difficult urination (dysuria) improved. Improvement occurred for only 9 of 17 women suffering from urinary frequency and 6 of 13 suffering from urinary urgency. These results were similar to those of a previous study, which demonstrated significant symptomatic relief in 80% of the 159 women studied who did not have bacteria present in their urine.[14]

There is one more advantage to alkalinizing, rather than acidifying, the urine. Many of the plant-based medicines used to treat urinary tract infections, such as goldenseal and uva-ursi, contain antibacterial components that work most effectively in an alkaline environment.

Rather than using potassium or sodium citrate alone, perhaps the best method of alkalinizing the urine is to take a multimineral formula in which the minerals are chelated to citrate or some other component of the Krebs cycle (such as malate, fumarate, or succinate). For example, in my clinical practice I typically recommend that women with bladder infections take 2 tablets of Krebs Cycle Chelates, a product made by Enzymatic Therapy, three times a day. This formula or similar formulas are usually available at health food stores.

Use Plant-Based Medicines

Many plants have been used through the centuries in the treatment of urinary tract infections. The two with the greatest scientific support for their use are uva-ursi and goldenseal.

Uva-Ursi　Other names for uva-ursi (*Archtostaphylos uva-ursi*) are bearberry and upland cranberry. Most research on uva-ursi's antiseptic properties for the urinary tract has focused on arbutin, which typically composes 7% to 9% of the leaves. However, crude plant extracts are much more medicinally effective than isolated arbutin.[15] Uva-ursi is reported to be especially active against *E. coli,* and it also has diuretic properties.[16,17]

Take care to avoid excessive dosages of uva-ursi. As little as 15 grams (½ ounce) of the dried leaves has produced toxicity in susceptible individuals. Signs of toxicity include ringing in the ears, nausea, vomiting, a sense of suffocation, shortness of breath, convulsions, delirium, and collapse.

Dosage (take these amounts, three times daily)

Dried leaves or as tea	1.5 to 4.0 grams (1 to 2 teaspoons in 8 ounces of hot water)
Tincture (1:5)	4 to 6 milliliters (1 to 1½ teaspoons)
Fluid extract (1:1)	0.5 to 2.0 milliliters (¼ to ½ teaspoon)
Powdered solid extract (10% arbutin content)	250 to 500 milligrams

Goldenseal   One of the most effective of botanical anti-microbial agents, goldenseal (*Hydrastis canadensis*) has a long history. Herbalists and naturopathic physicians continue to use it in the treatment of infections. Of particular importance is its efficacy against most common bacterial causes of bladder infections, including *E. coli.*[18] Goldenseal works best in an alkaline urine.

Dosage (take these amounts, three times daily)

Dried root or as tea	1 to 2 grams (1 to 2 teaspoons in 8 ounces of hot water)
Tincture (1:5)	4 to 6 milliliters (1 to 1½ teaspoons)

Fluid extract (1:1)	0.5 to 2.0 milliliters (¼ to ½ teaspoon)
Powdered solid extract (8% alkaloid content)	250–500 milligrams

Final Comments

Although most bladder infections are relatively benign, it is extremely important that they are properly diagnosed, treated, and monitored. Proper monitoring includes notifying a physician of any change in the condition. If a urine culture is positive for bacteria, it is appropriate to follow up with another culture 7 to 14 days after treatment begins.

For most bladder infections, the best treatment appears to be the natural approach. There is a growing concern that antibiotic therapy actually promotes recurrent bladder infections by disturbing the bacterial flora of the vagina. Antibiotic therapy may also lead to antibiotic-resistant strains of *E. coli*.[19,20] If antibiotics have been used, reintroduce "friendly" bacteria into the vagina. The best way to do this is to use products that contain active *Lactobacillus acidophilus*. These products are available at health food stores. Simply place 1 or 2 *Lactobacillus acidophilus* capsules or tablets in the vagina before going to bed.

Here is a concise treatment summary of the natural approach to bladder infections:

- Drink large amounts of fluids (at least 2 quarts per day), including at least 16 ounces of unsweetened cranberry or blueberry juice per day.
- Urinate after intercourse. A woman with a history of developing bladder infections after intercourse should wash her labia and urethra with strong goldenseal tea (2 teaspoons per cup) both before and after intercourse.

- Avoid all simple sugars, refined carbohydrates, full-strength fruit juice (diluted fruit juice is acceptable), and food allergens.
- Take 500 milligrams of vitamin C every 2 hours.
- Use either uva-ursi or goldenseal at the appropriate dosage.

5

Cold Hands and Feet

Cold hands and feet are common to women in general, not just menopausal women. In most instances, there are three major causes of cold hands and feet: hypothyroidism, low iron levels in the body, and poor circulation. Some detective work is needed to determine which factor is responsible in each case. Once the cause is identified, the treatment is straightforward.

Hypothyroidism

Much controversy surrounds the diagnosis of hypothyroidism. Before the components of the blood could be measured accurately, the diagnosis of hypothyroidism was based on basal body temperature (the temperature of the body at rest) and Achilles tendon reflex time (hypothyroidism slows the reflexes). With the advent of sophisticated laboratory measurement of thyroid hormones in the blood, these tests of thyroid function fell by the wayside. However, it is now known that blood tests are not sensitive enough to diagnose mild forms of hypothyroidism. Because mild hypothyroidism is the most common form, the majority of people with hypothyroidism are going undiagnosed.

The basal body temperature is perhaps the most sensitive indicator of thyroid function. A simple method for taking your basal body temperature follows.

Basal Body Temperature

Your body temperature reflects your metabolic rate, which is largely determined by hormones secreted by the thyroid gland. Therefore, by simply knowing your basal temperature, you and your physician can get an idea of how well your thyroid gland is functioning. All you need is a thermometer.

Taking Your Basal Body Temperature   Women who are still menstruating must perform the test on the second, third, and fourth days of menstruation. Postmenopausal women can perform the test upon waking at any time of the month.

   Procedure
   1. Shake down the thermometer to below 95 degrees Fahrenheit and place it by your bed before going to sleep at night.
   2. On waking, place the thermometer in your armpit for a full 10 minutes. Move as little as possible. Lie still and rest with your eyes closed. Do not get up until the 10-minute test is completed.
   3. After 10 minutes, read and record the temperature and date.
   4. Record the temperature for at least three mornings (preferably at the same time of day), and give the information to your physician.

Interpreting Your Basal Body Temperature   Your basal body temperature should be between 97.6 and 98.2 degrees

Fahrenheit. Low basal body temperatures are quite common and may reflect hypothyroidism. Other common signs and symptoms of hypothyroidism, in addition to cold hands and feet, are depression, difficulty in losing weight, dry skin, headaches, lethargy or fatigue, menstrual problems, recurrent infections, constipation, and sensitivity to cold.

High basal body temperatures (above 98.6 degrees) are less common than low body temperatures, but they may be evidence of hyperthyroidism. Common signs and symptoms of hyperthyroidism include bulging eyeballs, fast pulse, hyperactivity, inability to gain weight, insomnia, irritability, menstrual problems, and nervousness.

How Common Is Hypothyroidism?

Most estimates on the incidence of hypothyroidism are based on the incidence of low levels of thyroid hormone in the blood. As already mentioned, this may mean a large number of people with mild hypothyroidism go undetected. Nonetheless, using blood levels of thyroid hormones as the criteria, researchers estimate that between 1% and 4% of the adult population have moderate to severe hypothyroidism. According to estimates, another 10% to 12% have mild hypothyroidism. The rate of hypothyroidism increases steadily with advancing age.

Some writers of popular books estimate the rate of hypothyroidism in the general adult population to be approximately 40%. These writers use medical history, physical examination, and basal body temperatures along with blood thyroid levels as the diagnostic criteria.[1,2] It is likely that, using these criteria, the true rate of hypothyroidism is somewhere near 25% of the population.

Dietary Considerations in Hypothyroidism

The manufacture of thyroid hormones within the thyroid gland is dependent on several important nutrients. Deficiency of any of a number of vitamins and minerals, especially iodine, or ingestion of certain foods could result in hypo-thyroidism.

Thyroid hormones, such as thyroxine, are made from iodine and the amino acid tyrosine. When the level of iodine is low in the diet and blood, the cells of the thyroid gland may become quite large and form a goiter. A goiter is an enlarged thyroid gland.

Goiter is estimated to affect over 200 million people the world over. In all but 4% of these cases, the goiter is caused by an iodine deficiency. Because of the addition of iodine to table salt, iodine deficiency is now quite rare in the United States and other industrialized countries. (Iodine was first added to table salt in Michigan, where in 1924 the goiter rate was an incredible 47%.)

Few people in the United States are now considered iodine deficient, yet the rate of goiter is still relatively high (5% to 6%) in certain high-risk areas. People in these areas who suffer from goiter probably ingest certain foods that block iodine utilization. These foods are known as goitro-gens. Turnips, cabbage, mustard, cassava root, soybeans, peanuts, pine nuts, and millet are goitrogens. Cooking usually inactivates the mechanisms in these foods that block iodine utilization.

The recommended dietary allowance (RDA) for iodine in adults is quite small, 150 micrograms. Seafoods—includ-ing seaweeds such as kelp, as well as clams, lobsters, oysters, sardines, and other saltwater fish—are nature's richest sources of iodine. However, the majority of iodine is derived from the use of iodized salt (70 micrograms of iodine per gram of salt). Sea salt has little iodine. The average intake of iodine in the United States is estimated to be over 600 micrograms per day.

Too much iodine can actually inhibit thyroid gland synthesis. For this reason and because the only function of iodine in the body is for thyroid hormone synthesis, it is recommended that intake of iodine, through diet and supplementation, not exceed 1 milligram (1,000 micrograms) per day for any length of time.

Correction of Hypothyroidism

The medical treatment of hypothyroidism, in all but the mildest forms of the disease, involves the use of desiccated thyroid or synthetic thyroid hormone. Although synthetic hormones have become popular, many physicians (particularly naturopathic physicians) still prefer the use of desiccated natural thyroid, complete with all thyroid hormones.

The Food and Drug Administration (FDA) requires that the thyroid extracts sold in health food stores be "thyroxine-free." However, it is nearly impossible to remove all the hormone from the gland. In other words, think of health food store thyroid preparations as mild forms of desiccated natural thyroid. If you have mild hypothyroidism, these preparations may provide enough support to help you with your thyroid problem.

Since it is important to support the thyroid gland nutritionally by ensuring adequate intake of key nutrients required in the manufacture of thyroid hormone, most health food store thyroid products also contain supportive nutrients such as iodine, zinc, and tyrosine.

The dosage of commercial thyroid preparations really depends on the potency and level of supportive nutrients. Obviously, these factors vary from one manufacturer to the next. Therefore, it is best to follow the manufacturer's recommendations as provided on the product label. Use your basal body temperature to determine the effectiveness of the product.

Low Iron Levels

Low iron levels are linked to cold hands and feet. This symptom reflects the central role of iron in the hemoglobin molecule of red blood cells. The red blood cells, with the help of hemoglobin, transport oxygen from lungs to body tissues and transport carbon dioxide from tissues to lungs.

Iron deficiency is the most common cause of anemia, a condition in which the blood is deficient in red blood cells or the hemoglobin (iron-containing) portion of red blood cells. The symptoms of anemia, such as extreme fatigue, reflect a lack of oxygen in tissues and a buildup of carbon dioxide. If a person is anemic, their hands and feet are almost always cold.

If you suffer from cold hands and feet, have your physician perform a routine blood analysis (a complete blood cell count with hemoglobin levels) as well as measure the level of ferritin, an iron-containing protein in the blood. Realize that anemia is the last stage of iron deficiency. Routine blood analysis is not accurate enough for the diagnosis of iron deficiency that has not reached the stage of anemia.

In addition to cold hands and feet, low iron can also lead to fatigue and lack of endurance. Several researchers have clearly demonstrated that even slight iron-deficiency anemia leads to fatigue and a reduction in physical work capacity and productivity.[3,4] Impaired physical performance due to iron deficiency is not dependent on anemia.[5] The iron-dependent enzymes involved in energy production and metabolism will be impaired long before anemia occurs.

Dietary Sources of Iron

There are two forms of dietary iron: heme iron and non-heme iron. Heme iron is iron bound to hemoglobin and myoglobin. It is the most efficiently absorbed form of iron, with an approximate absorption rate of 25%.[6] Nonheme iron is poorly absorbed; its approximate absorption rate is 5%.

Heme iron is absorbed intact; nonheme iron must be ionized by stomach acid and be transported by complex

Table 5.1 Dietary Sources of Iron

Food	Average Serving Size (g)	Iron/Serving (mg)
Liver, calf or lamb	60	9.6
Liver, beef or chicken	60	5.2
Beef (meat)	90	2.7
Beans, cooked	100	2.3
Prunes	100	1.8
Bread, whole-grain enriched (3 slices)	70	1.7
Chicken or turkey (meat)	90	1.6
Greens, cooked	75	1.5
Peas	75	1.5
Eggs	50	1.1

mechanisms before it can be absorbed. Lack of stomach acid makes it difficult for many postmenopausal women to absorb iron and calcium.[7] In addition, nonheme iron is extremely susceptible to blocking agents such as fiber, phosphates, calcium, tannates, and preservatives.

Dietary sources of heme iron are animal meats, egg yolks, fish, and shellfish. As Table 5.1 shows, liver is regarded as the best dietary source of iron; it has a high heme iron content. Dietary sources of nonheme iron include beans, molasses, dried fruits, whole grain and enriched breads, and green leafy vegetables. Vitamin C enhances the absorption of nonheme iron.

Iron Supplements

Iron supplementation is often required to build up iron levels. Liver extracts provide the best form of iron—heme iron—and are therefore considered the best iron supplements. In addition, liver extracts contain other substances that promote healthy red blood cells. Many commercially available liver extracts provide the benefit of heme iron without the calories and fat that would accompany a similar amount of heme iron gained by eating liver or meat. If you are iron deficient, take two 500-milligram tablets or capsules of liver extract with your meals.

Despite the superiority of heme iron, nonheme iron salts are the most popular iron supplements. One reason: Even though heme iron is better absorbed, it is easy to take higher quantities of nonheme iron salts so that the net amount of iron absorbed is about equal. In other words, if you take 3 milligrams of heme iron and 50 milligrams of nonheme iron, the net absorption of each will be about the same.

Ferrous sulfate is the most popular iron salt in use, but it is among the least well tolerated. Gastrointestinal upset, nausea, and constipation or diarrhea are common complaints from those who use ferrous sulfate. Better-tolerated and better-absorbed forms of nonheme iron include iron bound to succinate, fumarate, ascorbate, glycinate, or apartate. The typical absorption rate for these iron salts is 2.9% on an empty stomach or 0.9% with food.[6] Physicians often recommend that iron salts be taken with food—this reduces such side effects as nausea, abdominal pain, and diarrhea. Unfortunately, taking the nonheme iron supplement with food greatly reduces its absorption. In contrast, the absorption rate of heme iron can be as high as 35% and is not affected by food.

If you are iron deficient and want to take a nonheme source, take 30 milligrams of iron, bound to either succinate or fumarate, twice daily, between meals. If this recommendation results in abdominal discomfort, take 30 milligrams with meals, three times daily.

In my clinical practice, I tend to recommend both heme and nonheme iron in the form of Enzymatic Therapy's Ultimate Iron. Each capsule contains 30 milligrams of ferrous succinate along with 250 milligrams of liquid liver fractions, a rich source of heme iron. In addition, Ultimate Iron provides other blood-building factors: vitamin C, folic acid, vitamin B12, and fat-soluble chlorophyll. If you want to use this formula, take 1 capsule twice daily, between meals, or 1 capsule with meals, three times daily.

Poor Circulation

Poor circulation is often due to atherosclerosis, or hardening of the arteries. Chapter 10 will discuss this topic in detail. The first step in improving blood flow through the hands and feet is to follow the recommendations in Chapter 10. These recommendations provide a long-term approach to the problem. To provide quicker benefits, use an extract of the leaves of *Ginkgo biloba*.

Ginkgo biloba is the world's oldest living tree species. From the dating of fossils containing ginkgo, it can be traced back more than 200 million years. For this reason, ginkgo is often referred to as the living fossil. Once common in North America and Europe, the Ice Age nearly destroyed ginkgo in all regions of the world except China. In China, it has long been cultivated as a sacred tree. Ginkgo is now grown throughout much of the United States. It is frequently planted along streets in cities because it is resistant to insects, disease, and pollution.

The medicinal use of *Ginkgo biloba* can be traced back to the oldest Chinese *materia medica* (2800 B.C.). The ginkgo leaves have been used in traditional Chinese medicine for their ability to "benefit the brain." As the next chapter will detail, ginkgo does indeed do just that. An extract of the leaves of the ginkgo tree is widely recommended in Europe to help improve the amount of blood flow to the brain. In fact, ginkgo extract is among the most popular medications in France and Germany.

In addition to improving blood flow to the brain, *Ginkgo biloba* extract exerts a number of beneficial effects on the vascular system and may prove to be helpful in treating hot flashes as well as cold hands and feet. *Ginkgo biloba* extract has improved blood flow to the hands and feet in human clinical trials and has been effective in the treatment of peripheral vascular disease of the extremities, including Raynaud's syndrome, a disease characterized by extremely cold fingers or toes.[8-10]

In order to take advantage of *ginkgo,* the product you use must be standardized to contain 24% ginkgo flavon-glycosides. The standard dosage of this extract is 40 milligrams, three times a day. Don't expect an immediate improvement. *Ginkgo biloba* extract will produce better results the longer it is used.

Final Comments

Hypothyroidism, low iron levels in the body, and poor circulation can cause more than cold hands and feet. Therefore, the recommendations in this chapter are appropriate for the treatment of many conditions, including impaired mental function, depression, and inability to concentrate.

6

Forgetfulness, Mental Distractedness, and Depression

Forgetfulness and the inability to concentrate are common symptoms of menopause. Often these symptoms are simply a result of a decreased supply of oxygen and nutrients to the brain. The brain is highly dependent on a constant supply of oxygen and nutrients. Although weighing only 3 pounds, the brain utilizes about 20% of the oxygen supply of the entire body. In dealing with the forgetfulness and mental concentration problems of menopause, the goal is to improve the supply of blood, oxygen, and nutrients to the brain.

Could Hypoglycemia Be a Factor?

The most critical nutrient for brain function is glucose, or blood sugar. The brain is dependent on glucose as an energy source. When the glucose level is low, as it is in cases of hypoglycemia (low blood sugar), the brain does not function properly. As a result, forgetfulness, lessened mental acuity, dizziness, headache, blurred vision, emotional instability, confusion, and abnormal behavior may occur.

How do you know if hypoglycemia is contributing to the forgetfulness of menopause? All things (especially cost) considered, the most useful way to diagnose hypoglycemia remains the assessment of symptoms. The hypoglycemia questionnaire (Figure 6.1) is an excellent tool for screening for hypoglycemia. If your score indicates hypoglycemia may be a factor, please consult *Diabetes and Hypolgycemia,* another book in the Getting Well Naturally series, and discuss hypoglycemia with your doctor.

No = 0   Mild = 1   Moderate = 2   Severe = 3

Crave sweets 0 1 2 3
Irritable if a meal is missed 0 1 2 3
Feel tired or weak if a meal is missed 0 1 2 3
Dizziness when standing suddenly 0 1 2 3
Frequent headaches 0 1 2 3
Poor memory (forgetful) or concentration 0 1 2 3
Feel tired an hour or so after eating 0 1 2 3
Heart palpitations 0 1 2 3
Feel shaky at times 0 1 2 3
Afternoon fatigue 0 1 2 3
Vision blurs on occasion 0 1 2 3
Depression or mood swings 0 1 2 3
Overweight 0 1 2 3
Frequently anxious or nervous 0 1 2 3
Total: _____

Scoring:

Less than 5 = Hypoglycemia is probably not a factor
6–15 = Hypoglycemia is a likely factor
Greater than 15 = Hypoglycemia is extremely likely

Figure 6.1   The hypoglycemia questionnaire

Nutrition, Blood Flow, and the Brain

The brain is so metabolically active that virtually every known vitamin and mineral is required for it to function properly. Many of these nutrients are utilized in the manufacture of important brain compounds, including neurotransmitters. Neurotransmitters are required for the transmission of information from nerve cell to nerve cell.[1]

Without an adequate level of any single nutrient, brain chemistry is altered. Nutritional deficiency could result not only in forgetfulness and impaired mental function, but also in depression, anxiety, and other mental disorders.[2] The best approach to ensure adequate levels of important vitamins and minerals is to follow the recommendations given in Chapter 12.

Most important, do what you can to ensure a good supply of blood and oxygen to the brain. Lack of blood flow to the brain, or cerebral vascular insufficiency, is an extremely common condition in the United States—this is due to the high rate of atherosclerosis among Americans (see Chapter 10). The atherosclerotic plaque pinches off the flow of blood to the brain. The major symptoms of cerebral vascular insufficiency are impaired mental performance, short-term memory loss, dizziness, headaches, ringing in the ears, and depression. These symptoms are extremely common in many postmenopausal women.

In addition to following the recommendations given in Chapter 10, use *Ginkgo biloba* extract to improve blood flow to the brain. As Chapter 5 discussed, in Europe an extract of the leaves of the ginkgo tree is widely recommended to help improve blood flow to the brain. In 1989, more than 100,000 physicians worldwide recommended ginkgo more than 10,000,000 times. *Ginkgo biloba* extract is one of the most popular plant-based products in America, as well.

There have been over 300 scientific studies to substantiate the ability of ginkgo to improve mental health.

A recent analysis assessed the quality of research in more than 40 clinical studies of a standardized extract of *Ginkgo biloba* leaves in the treatment of cerebral insufficiency.[3] The results indicated that the quality of the research was on a par with the research used to investigate ergoloid mesylates (Hydergine), a drug approved by the FDA in the treatment of dementia (including Alzheimer's disease). The analysis further substantiated that *Ginkgo biloba* extract is effective in reducing all symptoms of cerebral insufficiency, including impaired mental function and forgetfulness.

Ginkgo biloba extract appears to work not only by increasing blood flow to the brain, but also by enhancing energy production within the brain. It increases the uptake of glucose by brain cells and actually improves the transmission of nerve signals.[4] All these effects contribute equally to the positive effects noted by the millions of people worldwide who are taking ginkgo.

Improving the transmission rate of the nerve signal is critically important to memory. Memory is directly related to the speed at which the nerve impulse can be transmitted. The faster the impulse is transmitted, the better your memory is. Double-blind studies have shown that ginkgo can significantly improve memory in elderly as well as college-aged women.[5–8] Although the effect of *Ginkgo biloba* extract on forgetfulness caused by menopause has not been studied with controls in place, evidence from other studies indicates that using gingko for menopausal forgetfulness is worth a try.

To take advantage of ginkgo's effect on brain function, use the same extract that is available in Europe. The product should be standardized to contain 24% ginkgo flavonglycosides. (Other components are important in the pharmacological activity of ginkgo, including terpene molecules known as ginkgolides.) The standard dosage of the 24% ginkgo flavonglycoside extract is 40 milligrams, three times a day.

Ginkgo biloba extract is extremely safe to use; there have been no reports of significant adverse reactions at the prescribed dosage. Mild adverse reactions, although quite rare, include gastrointestinal upset and headache.

In the treatment of cerebral vascular insufficiency, take *Ginkgo biloba* extract consistently for at least 12 weeks to determine effectiveness in your case. Although most people report benefits within two to three weeks, some take longer to respond. It seems that the longer the treatment is continued, the more obvious and lasting the result.

Ginkgo biloba extract is showing great benefit in many cases of senility. In addition to the ability of the extract to increase the functional capacity of the brain, it also addresses many of the effects of Alzheimer's disease. Thus, gingko may help many people to maintain a normal life and escape nursing home care. At this time, however, studies indicate that *Ginkgo biloba* extract can help delay and possibly reverse the mental deterioration in only the early stages of Alzheimer's disease. However, if the mental deficit is due to vascular insufficiency or depression and not Alzheimer's disease, *Ginkgo biloba* extract will usually be effective in reversing the deficit.

Depression

Another complaint common to menopausal women is depression. Ginkgo does exert some antidepressant activity and may be helpful in this regard. Another plant to try is St. John's wort, a shrubby perennial native to many parts of the world, including Europe and the United States. Researchers in Europe have discovered that components of St. John's wort alter brain chemistry in a way that improves mood. These effects have been confirmed in clinical studies in which a standardized extract of St. John's wort (0.125% hypericin) led to significant improvement in symptoms of anxiety, depression, and feelings of worthlessness.[9] In fact, the effectiveness of the St. John's wort extract in relieving depression was greater than that produced by standard drugs used to treat depression, including amitriptyline (Elavil) and imipramine (Tofranil).[10] These drugs are associated with significant side effects (most often drowsiness, dry mouth, constipation, and impaired urination). St. John's wort extract, in contrast, is not associated with any significant side effect.

In addition to improving mood, the extract has been shown to greatly improve sleep quality, and it was effective in relieving both insomnia and hypersomnia. The dosage used in these studies has typically been 300 to 500 milligrams of the extract (0.125% hypericin), three times daily.

7

Maintenance of Healthy Bones

Osteoporosis literally means porous bone. Osteoporosis affects more than 20 million people in the United States. Normally, after the age of 40, bone mass declines in both sexes, but women are at a much greater risk for osteoporosis than are men. Many factors can result in excessive bone loss, and different variants of osteoporosis exist. Postmenopausal osteoporosis is the most common form, however. Approximately one in four postmenopausal women has osteoporosis.[1]

Although the entire skeleton may be involved in post-menopausal osteoporosis, bone loss is usually greatest in the spine, hips, and ribs. Since these bones bear a great deal of weight, those who suffer from osteoporosis are susceptible to pain, deformity, and fracture. At least 1.5 million fractures occur each year as a direct result of osteoporosis. Of these fractures, 250,000 are hip fractures, the most catastrophic of fractures. Hip fracture, which is fatal in 12% to 20% of cases, precipitates long-term nursing home care for half of those who survive. Nearly one-third of all women and one-sixth of all men will fracture their hips.

Certain conditions or characteristics predispose a woman to osteoporosis.

Major Risk Factors for Osteoporosis in Women
Postmenopausal status
White or Asian
Premature menopause
Positive family history of osteoporosis
Short stature and small bones
Leanness
Low calcium intake
Inactivity
Nulliparity (the status of never having been pregnant)
Gastric or small-bowel resection
Long-term glucocorticosteroid therapy
Long-term use of anticonvulsants
Hyperparathyroidism
Hyperthyroidism
Smoking
Heavy alcohol use

Osteoporosis involves both the mineral (inorganic) and the nonmineral components of bone. The nonmineral components constitute the organic matrix of bone, which is composed primarily of protein. That osteoporosis involves mineral and nonmineral deficiencies should tip you off to the fact that there is more to osteoporosis than a lack of dietary calcium. In fact, lack of dietary calcium in an adult results in a separate condition known as osteomalacia, or softening of the bone. In osteoporosis, in contrast, there is a lack of calcium and other minerals as well as a decrease in the nonmineral framework (organic matrix) of bone. Little attention has been given to the important role that this organic matrix plays in maintaining bone structure.

Calcium Metabolism and Hormonal Factors in Osteoporosis

Bone is dynamic living tissue that is constantly being broken down and rebuilt, even in adults. Normal bone metabolism is dependent on an intricate interplay of many nutritional and hormonal factors, with the liver and kidney having a regulatory effect. Although over two dozen nutrients are necessary for optimal bone health, it is generally thought that calcium and vitamin D are the most important. However, hormones are also critical. In women, the incorporation of calcium into bone is dependent upon the hormone estrogen.

To understand current theories about how osteoporosis develops, it is necessary to briefly examine normal calcium metabolism (absorption, storage, and excretion).

The Importance of Stomach Acid

To be absorbed, calcium must be ionized in the intestines. (The need for solubility and ionization has been the major problem with the most widely utilized form of calcium as a nutritional supplement, calcium carbonate.) Studies of postmenopausal women have shown that about 40% are severely deficient in stomach acid.[2] Patients with insufficient stomach acid can only absorb about 4% of an oral dose of calcium as calcium carbonate; a person with normal stomach acid can typically absorb about 22%.[3] Patients with low stomach acid secretion need a form of calcium already in a soluble and ionized state—a form such as calcium citrate, calcium lactate, or calcium gluconate. Patients with reduced stomach acid can absorb about 45% of the calcium from calcium citrate.[3]

Studies also demonstrate that, like those with low levels of stomach acid, normal subjects can absorb calcium from calcium citrate better than that from calcium carbonate.[4] In any event, in terms of absorbability, calcium citrate and other soluble forms (lactate, aspartate, orotate, and so on) appear to be the best calcium supplements at this time.

Vitamin D

It is well known that vitamin D stimulates the absorption of calcium. Since vitamin D can be produced in our bodies by the action of sunlight on 7-dihydroxycholesterol in the skin, many experts consider it more of a hormone than a vitamin. The sunlight changes the 7-dihydroxycholesterol into vitamin D3 (cholecalciferol). It is then transported to the liver and converted by an enzyme into 25-hydroxy-cholecalciferol ($25\text{-}OHD_3$), which is five times more potent than cholecalciferol. The 25-hydroxycholecalciferol is then converted by an enzyme in the kidneys to 1,25-dihydroxy-cholecalciferol ($1,25\text{-}(OH)_2D_3$), which is 10 times more potent than cholecalciferol and the most potent form of vitamin D3 (see Figure 7.1).

Disorders of the liver or kidneys result in impaired conversion of cholecalciferol to more potent vitamin D compounds. In many patients with osteoporosis, there are high levels of $25\text{-}OHD_3$ but the level of $1,25\text{-}(OH)_2D_3$ is quite low. This signifies an impairment of renal conversion of $25\text{-}OHD_3$ to $1,25\text{-}(OH)_2D_3$ in osteoporosis.[5,6] Many theories have been proposed to account for this decreased conversion, including relationships to estrogen and magnesium deficiency. Recently, some theories suggest that the trace mineral boron has a role in this conversion.

Hormonal Factors

The concentration of calcium in the blood is strictly maintained within very narrow limits. If the level starts

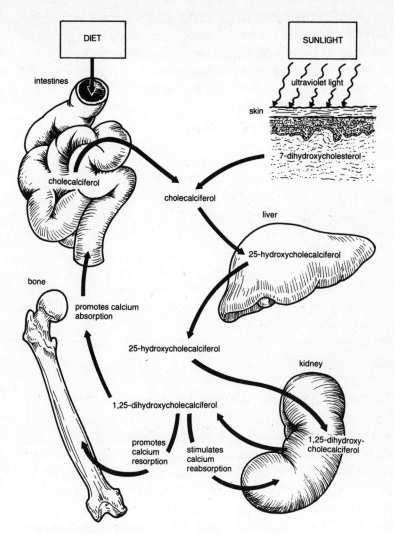

Figure 7.1   Vitamin D metabolism

to decrease, the parathyroid glands increase the secretion of parathyroid hormone and the thyroid and parathyroids decrease the secretion of calcitonin. If the calcium level in the blood starts to increase, there is a decrease in the secretion of parathyroid hormone and an increase in the secretion of calcitonin. To understand osteoporosis, it is necessary to understand how the parathyroid hormone increases and the hormone calcitonin decreases serum calcium.

Parathyroid hormone increases serum calcium primarily by increasing the activity of the cells that break down bone (osteoclasts). Also, it decreases the excretion of calcium by the kidneys and increases the absorption of calcium in the intestines. In the kidneys, parathyroid hormone increases the conversion of 25-OHD_3 to $1,25\text{-(OH)}_2\text{D}_3$.

One of the theories relating bone loss to estrogen deficiency maintains that an estrogen deficiency makes the osteoclasts more sensitive to parathyroid hormone. The result is increased bone breakdown and an increase in calcium in the blood. This elevation in blood calcium leads to a decreased parathyroid hormone level, which results in diminished levels of active vitamin D and increased calcium excretion as well. Evidence seems to support this theory.[5-7]

Dietary Considerations in Bone Health

Recently, there has been an incredible push for increasing dietary calcium to prevent osteoporosis. This appears to be sound medical advice for many. But, as you know, osteoporosis is much more than a lack of dietary calcium. It is a complex condition involving hormonal, lifestyle, nutrition, and environmental factors. A comprehensive plan that addresses these factors offers the greatest protection against developing osteoporosis.

The primary goals of a diet to treat and prevent osteoporosis are to (1) preserve adequate mineral mass, (2) prevent loss of the protein matrix and other structural components of bone, and (3) ensure optimal repair mechanisms to remodel damaged areas of bone.

General Dietary Factors

Many general dietary factors have been suggested as causes of osteoporosis: low-calcium, high-phosphorus intake; a high-protein diet; a high-acid, high-ash diet; and trace mineral deficiencies, to name a few. To help slow bone loss, foods high in calcium are often recommended. Besides dairy products, foods rich in calcium include kale, spinach, turnip greens, and other green leafy vegetables.

Compared to an omnivore's diet, a vegetarian's diet (both lacto-ovo and vegan) is associated with a lower risk of osteoporosis.[8,9] Although the bone mass of vegetarians does not differ significantly from that of omnivores in the third, fourth, and fifth decades, there are significant differences in the later decades. These findings indicate that the decreased incidence of osteoporosis in vegetarians is not due to increased initial bone mass, but decreased bone loss.

Several factors are probably responsible for the relatively small amount of bone loss in vegetarians. Most important: the lowered intake of protein. A high-protein diet or a diet high in phosphates increases the excretion of calcium in the urine. Raising daily protein from 47 to 142 grams doubles the excretion of calcium in the urine.[10] A diet this high in protein is common in the United States and may be a significant factor in the increased number of people suffering from osteoporosis in this country.

Another dietary factor that increases the loss of calcium from the body is refined sugar. After sugar intake, there is an increase in the urinary excretion of calcium.[11] Consider that the average American consumes, in one day, 150 grams of sucrose plus other refined simple sugars, a glass of a carbonated beverage loaded with phosphates, and a large amount of protein. It is little wonder that so many Americans suffer from osteoporosis. When lifestyle factors are taken into consideration, it is very apparent why osteoporosis has become a major medical problem.

The Importance of Green Leafy Vegetables

Green leafy vegetables (kale, collard greens, parsley, lettuce, and so on) offer significant protection against osteoporosis. These foods are a rich source of a broad range of vitamins and minerals important to maintaining healthy bones: calcium, vitamin K1, and boron are among the most important.

Vitamin K1 is the form of vitamin K that is found in plants. A function of vitamin K1 that is often overlooked is its role in converting inactive osteocalcin to its active form. Osteocalcin is the major noncollagen protein in bone. Its role in bone is to anchor calcium molecules within the bone.

A deficiency of vitamin K leads to impaired mineralization of bone due to inadequate osteocalcin levels. Very low blood levels of vitamin K1 have been found in patients with fractures due to osteoporosis.[12] The severity of fracture strongly correlates with the level of circulating vitamin K. The lower the level of vitamin K, the greater the severity of the fracture. Since vitamin K is found in green leafy vegetables, it may be one of the key reasons why vegetarian diet offers protection against osteoporosis.

The high levels of minerals such as calcium and boron in green leafy vegetables may also be responsible for this protective effect. Boron is a trace mineral that has gained recent attention as a protective factor against osteoporosis.[13] Supplementing the diet of postmenopausal women with 3 milligrams of boron per day reduced urinary calcium excretion by 44% and dramatically increased the levels of 17-beta-estradiol, the most biologically active estrogen.[13] Boron seems to activate certain hormones, including estrogen and vitamin D. You already know that vitamin D is converted to its most active form $(1,25\text{-}(OH)_2D_3)$ within the kidney and that this conversion is impaired in postmenopausal osteoporosis. Boron is apparently required for this reaction to occur. A boron deficiency may contribute greatly to osteoporosis as well as menopausal symptoms.

Fruits and vegetables are the main dietary sources of boron, so diets low in these foods may be deficient in boron. Typically, the standard American diet is severely deficient in these foods. According to several large surveys, including the U.S. Second National Health and Nutrition Examination, fewer than 10% of Americans meet the minimum recommendation of 2 fruit servings and 3 vegetable servings per day. Only 51% eat 1 serving of vegetables per day.[14]

To guarantee adequate boron intake, supplement the diet with a daily dose of 3 to 5 milligrams of boron. Boron has been shown to mimic some of the effects of estrogen therapy in postmenopausal women.[15]

Nutritional Supplementation for Bone Health

Bone is dependent on a constant supply of many nutrients. A deficiency of any one of these will adversely affect bone health. In addition to vitamin K and boron, here is a brief discussion of nutrients critical to bone health and guidelines about supplementing your diet with them.

Calcium

Supplementation with calcium has been shown to be effective in reducing bone loss in postmenopausal women.[1,16,17] Many experts are recommending a daily calcium intake of 1,500 milligrams. This typically means that supplementation in the range of 1,000 to 1,200 milligrams is required. As mentioned, the absorption and retention of calcium is dependent on a complex interplay of hormones and other factors. The initial approach is supplementation with the most bioavailable form of calcium. At this time, calcium citrate appears to be the best form of calcium, in terms of absorption and risk of kidney stone development.[3,4,18]

Some are concerned that increased calcium supplementation may result in increased calcium oxalate kidney stones. Calcium citrate appears not to warrant this concern. Though the level of urinary calcium rises in patients consuming calcium citrate, citrate inhibits the formation of kidney stones. Specifically, citrate reduces urinary saturation of calcium oxalate and calcium phosphate and retards the nucleation and crystal growth of calcium salts.[18,19] The use of potassium or sodium citrate in the treatment of recurrent calcium oxalate has been shown to be quite effective in clinical studies. Stone formation ceased in nearly 90% of the subjects.[17] In the future, magnesium citráte may prove to be the citrate of choice in the treatment of recurrent calcium oxalate kidney stones. Magnesium seems to have the ability to increase the solubility of calcium oxalate and inhibit the precipitation of both calcium phosphate and calcium oxalate.[20]

Other Krebs cycle intermediates—such as fumarate, malate, succinate, and aspartate—can be used in combination with citrate. Generally, over 95% of the Krebs cycle intermediates ingested are used as energy substrates; the remainder are excreted in the urine. Thus, the Krebs cycle intermediates fulfill every requirement for an agent that combines optimally with calcium: They are easily ionized, they are almost completely degraded, they are virtually nontoxic, and they may increase the absorption of calcium and other minerals.

Magnesium

Magnesium supplementation is apparently as important as calcium supplementation. The bones of women with osteoporosis have a lower magnesium content than those of people without osteoporosis, and women with osteoporosis show other signs of magnesium deficiency.[21] In human magnesium deficiency, there is a decrease in serum concentration of the most active form of vitamin D (1,25-$(OH)_2D_3$). A low level of this form has been observed in osteoporosis.[22] This could be due to the fact that the enzyme responsible for the conversion of 25-OHD$_3$ to 1,25-(OH)$_2$D$_3$ is dependent on adequate magnesium. Or, it could reflect the ability of magnesium to mediate parathyroid hormone and calcitonin secretion.

Intake of dairy foods fortified with vitamin D results in decreased magnesium absorption.[23] This effect, combined with the fact that a high number of women with osteoporosis cannot tolerate milk (27% to 47%), indicates that milk may not be an appropriate food to prevent osteoporosis.[24]

Vitamin B6, Folic Acid, and Vitamin B12

Low levels of these nutrients are quite common in the elderly population. Their lack may contribute to osteoporosis.[17,25] These vitamins are important in the conversion of the amino acid methionine to cysteine. A deficiency of these vitamins or a defect in the enzymes responsible for methionine conversion leads to an increase in homocysteine. This compound has been implicated in a variety of conditions, including atherosclerosis and osteoporosis.

Increased homocysteine concentrations in the blood are associated with postmenopausal women and are thought to play a role in osteoporosis by interfering with collagen cross-linking. The result is a defective bone matrix. Since osteoporosis is known to be a loss of both the organic and inorganic phases of bone, the homocysteine theory may have much validity, in that it is one of the few theories that addresses both factors.

Folic acid supplementation has reduced homocysteine levels in postmenopausal women, even though none of the women were deficient in folic acid according to standard laboratory criteria.

Vitamin B6 and B12 are also necessary in the metabolism of homocysteine. A diet deficient in vitamin B6 produces osteoporosis in rats, a result that demonstrates the importance of vitamin B6 in bone health.

Silicon

Silicon is responsible for cross-linking the collagen strands. Therefore, silicon contributes greatly to the strength and integrity of the connective tissue matrix of bone.[17] Since silicon concentrations are increased at calcification sites in growing bone, recalcification in bone remodeling may be dependent on adequate levels of silicon. It is not known whether the typical American diet provides adequate amounts of silicon. In patients with osteoporosis or where accelerated bone regeneration is desired, silicon requirements may be increased; therefore, supplementation may be indicated.

The Importance of Lifestyle

Certain lifestyle factors are extremely important to bone health. For example, the use of coffee, alcohol, and tobacco induce a negative calcium balance and are associated with an increased risk of developing osteoporosis; regular exercise reduces the risk.[17,26] In fact, as important as hormonal and dietary factors are, they are not the most critical factors for maintaining healthy bones. Exercise is the most critical.

Numerous studies have clearly demonstrated that physical fitness is the major determinant of bone density. Physical exercise consisting of one hour of moderate activity three times a week has been shown to prevent bone loss and actually increase bone mass in postmenopausal women.[17,27–30] In contrast to exercise, immobilization doubles the rate of urinary and fecal calcium excretion, which results in a significant negative calcium balance.[31]

If you are interested in learning more about osteoporosis, I strongly encourage you to read *Preventing and Reversing Osteoporosis* by Alan R. Gaby, M.D. (Prima Publishing, Rocklin, CA, 1994).

8

Prevention of Breast Cancer

Breast cancer is a serious medical concern for women. Current estimates state that one woman in nine will develop breast cancer. Each year roughly 175,000 new cases of breast cancer are diagnosed and 50,000 women will die of breast cancer. The survival rate for women with breast cancer has not been significantly improved with modern surgical, radiation, or chemotherapy. Therefore, the best treatment for breast cancer is prevention.

Are you at risk for breast cancer? Consider the list that follows.

Risk Factors for Breast Cancer
Advancing age
Family history of breast cancer
High intake of animal fat
First baby born after age 30
Never been pregnant
Early start of menses

Excessive exposure to radiation
Regular alcohol consumption
History of fibrocystic breast disease
History of oral contraceptive use or estrogen replacement therapy

Prevention of breast cancer involves reducing controllable risk factors. Obviously, you cannot choose new biological parents to obviate a family history of breast cancer, but you can employ measures to significantly reduce your risk of breast cancer. The major controllable risk factor for breast cancer is diet.

Diet in the Prevention of Breast Cancer

While the incidence of breast cancer is reaching epidemic proportions in the United States, in other parts of the world it is quite low. Is diet the reason? Definitely. Americans simply consume more fat, cholesterol, animal protein, and sugar and eat fewer vegetables, fruits, whole grains, and legumes than people in most other societies.[1] As a result, chronic degenerative diseases like breast cancer, heart disease, diabetes, and stroke are extremely common in America. To illustrate the importance of diet in the prevention of breast cancer, let's examine some interesting population studies.

Perhaps the most interesting tried to figure out why Japanese women are only one-fifth as likely to develop breast cancer as American women. Are genetic factors responsible? The answer appears to be no because, when Japanese women move to the United States and adopt American eating habits, their risk of breast cancer eventually reaches that of American women.[1,2]

The traditional Japanese diet is much different than the standard American diet. In Japan, only 20% of the calories in the daily diet come from fat, compared to 40% in the United States. Also, the Japanese diet is rich in soy foods, fish, cabbage-family vegetables, and garlic. All these foods exert a protective effect against breast cancer. Obviously, if American women want to significantly reduce their risk of breast cancer, they need to alter their diets to reduce risk.

Dietary Fats and Breast Cancer

Breast cancer is associated with a diet high in animal fats.[1,3] Therefore, the first step in reducing your risk of breast cancer is simply to reduce the amount of animal fats in your diet. As a bonus, this will also reduce your risk of developing other cancers as well as heart disease.[1] To see why, take a closer look at dietary fats.

Animal fats are typically solid at room temperature and are referred to as saturated fats. Vegetable fats are liquid at room temperature and are referred to as unsaturated fats or oils. Our bodies need certain types of fats known as essential fatty acids. The two essential fatty acids are linoleic acid and linolenic acid. These fatty acids function in our bodies as components of nerve cells, cellular membranes, and hormonelike substances known as prostaglandins. Essential fatty acids are critical to normal body function and also lower cholesterol and protect against athero-sclerosis. Most vegetable oils are a good source of essential fatty acids. In contrast, most animal fats contain relatively small amounts of essential fatty acids. Instead, animal fats are composed primarily of saturated fats and cholesterol.

Although our bodies require essential fatty acids, too much fat in the diet, especially saturated fat, is linked to numerous cancers, including breast cancer, as well as heart disease and stroke.[1] Most nutrition experts recommend that total fat intake be kept below 30% of total calories. However, to significantly reduce the risk of breast cancer, it may be necessary to reduce the amount of fat to below 20% of total calories, especially for women with a history of breast cancer.[4] Experts also recommend consuming at least twice as much unsaturated fat as saturated fat. This recommendation is easy to follow: Simply reduce the amount of animal products in the diet; use natural polyunsaturated oils such as canola, safflower, soy, and flaxseed; and consume more nuts and seeds.

Most commercially available salad dressings, as well as those in restaurants, are full of the wrong type of fats and oils. Salad dressings are the perfect opportunity to use polyunsaturated and therapeutic vegetable oils. In *The Healing Power of Foods Cookbook* (Prima Publishing, Rocklin, CA, 1993), I give recipes for salad dressings. You will find a recipe for Herb Dressing in Chapter 11.

The best vegetable oil to use is flaxseed oil. Flaxseeds are the most abundant source of lignans. Lignans—compounds found in seeds, grains, and legumes—provide anticancer, antibacterial, antifungal, and antiviral activity.[5] Plant lignans are changed, by flora in the gut, into enterolactone and enterodiol, two compounds believed to be particularly protective against breast cancer. Experiments in which animals were fed high-lignan diets showed that lignans provide tremendous protection against mammary cancer. Lignans are thought to be one of the reasons for the low rate of breast cancer in vegetarian women.[6]

In addition to lignans, flaxseed oil is also rich in linolenic acid, an omega-3 oil.[7] Omega-3 oils from fish have shown impressive anticancer effects in animal experiments, and fish consumption has been shown to be protective against breast cancer (presumably because of the omega-3 oil content). Look for flaxseed oils, like Barlean's, that are rich in lignan. (Barlean's is available at most health food stores.)

Fats and Oils to Avoid   In addition to animal fats, certain vegetable fats and oils are best avoided. At the top of the list are margarine and shortening. During the process of margarine and shortening manufacture, vegetable oils are hydrogenated. This means that a hydrogen molecule is added to the natural unsaturated fatty-acid molecules of the vegetable oil. Hydrogenation changes the structure of the natural fatty acid. The result is a vegetable oil that is solid or semisolid.

Many researchers and nutritionists have been concerned about the health effects of margarine since it was first introduced. Although many Americans assume they are doing their body good by consuming margarine instead of butter and saturated fats, in truth they are actually doing harm. Population studies indicate that margarine and shortening use is a significant risk factor for breast cancer, even in low-risk women.[8] In addition, studies show that margarine and other hydrogenated vegetable oils increase the risk for heart disease. They not only raise LDL cholesterol, but they also lower the protective HDL cholesterol level, interfere with essential fatty-acid metabolism, and are suspected of causing certain cancers.[8,9] If you desire a butterlike spread, use a canola oil product that is not hydrogenated.

In addition to margarine and shortening, do not use cottonseed, coconut, or palm oil. These oils are primarily saturated fat and they may contain toxic residues.

Fruits and Vegetables

Fruit and vegetable consumption has been associated with a reduced risk for many cancers, including breast cancer.[1,2,10,11] Fruits and vegetables are rich sources of many beneficial anticancer compounds, including vitamin C, carotenes, flavonoids, and trace minerals. These compounds are known as antioxidants because they can protect against damage produced by highly reactive molecules that bind to and destroy cellular components. These highly reactive compounds are called free radicals, or pro-oxidants. Free radical damage is what makes us age. It also initiates the development of many other diseases: cancer, heart disease, cataracts, Alzheimer's disease, and virtually every other chronic degenerative disease.

Although the body creates free radicals during metabolism, the environment contributes greatly to an individual's free radical load. Cigarette smoking, for example, greatly increases the free radical load. Many of the harmful effects of smoking are related to the extremely high levels of free radicals that are inhaled. The free radicals deplete key antioxidant nutrients, such as vitamin C and beta-carotene. Other external sources of free radicals include ionizing radiation, air pollutants, pesticides, anesthetics, aromatic hydrocarbons, fried food, solvents, alcohol, and formaldehyde. These compounds greatly stress the body's antioxidant mechanisms and should be avoided as much as possible.

Although all the antioxidant nutrients from plants are important in preventing breast cancer, research indicates that carotene and vitamin C are the most important. Studies have consistently demonstrated an inverse relationship between the intake of these nutrients and cancer incidence: The higher the intake of vitamin C or carotenes, the lower the incidence of most cancers.

Carotenes, or carotenoids, represent the most widespread group of naturally occurring pigments in nature. They are a highly colored (red to yellow) group of fat-soluble compounds that protect plants against damage produced during photosynthesis. Carotenes are best known for their capacity to convert into vitamin A and for their antioxidant activity.

Over 400 carotenes have been characterized, but only 30 to 50 are believed to have vitamin A activity. These are referred to as provitamin A carotenes. The biological effects of a carotene are usually attributed to its vitamin A activity. In fact, beta-carotene has been considered the most active of the carotenes, because its provitamin A activity is higher than that of other carotenes. However, recent research suggests that these vitamin A activities have been over-emphasized; other, non–vitamin A carotenes exhibit far greater antioxidant and anticancer effects.[12-14]

Unlike vitamin A, which is stored primarily in the liver, unconverted carotenes are stored in fat cells, epithelial cells, and other organs (the adrenals, testes, and ovaries have the highest concentrations). Epithelial cells are found in the skin and the linings of our internal organs (including the respiratory tract, gastrointestinal tract, and genitourinary tract). Population studies have demonstrated a strong correlation between carotene intake and a variety of cancers involving epithelial tissues (lung, skin, uterine cervix, gastrointestinal tract, and so on).[1,2,10] The higher the carotene intake, the lower the risk of cancer. Scientific studies are also showing that carotenes have antitumor and immune-enhancing effects.[13,14]

Another difference between vitamin A and carotenes is that too much vitamin A can be toxic. In contrast, you cannot consume too many carotenes. Studies of beta-carotene show it to have no significant toxicity, even when used in very high doses in the treatment of medical conditions.[15] High carotene consumption can, however, result in the appearance of slightly yellow to orange skin. This is due to the storage of carotenes in epithelial cells, and the condition is known as carotenodermia. It is nothing to be alarmed about. In fact, it is probably a sign that the body has a good supply of carotenes.

The leading sources of carotenes are dark-green leafy vegetables (kale, collards, and spinach) and yellow-orange fruits and vegetables (apricots, cantaloupe, carrots, sweet potatoes, yams, and squash). The carotenes present in green plants are found in the chloroplasts, with chlorophyll—usually in complexes with a protein or lipid. Beta-carotene is the predominant carotene form in most green leaves. In general, the greater the intensity of the green color, the greater the concentration of beta-carotene.

Orange-colored fruits and vegetables (carrots, apricots, mangoes, yams, squash, and so on) typically have higher concentrations of provitamin A carotenes than beta-carotene. The provitamin A content parallels the intensity of the color.

In the orange and yellow fruits and vegetables, beta-carotene concentrations are high, but other carotenes are present as well. These include many with antioxidant and anticancer effects that are more potent than those of beta-carotene. The red and purple vegetables and fruits (such as tomatoes, red cabbage, berries, and plums) contain significant amounts of carotenes; legumes, grains, and seeds are also valuable sources of carotenes.[16]

Eat carotene-rich foods regularly. Most of these foods are also excellent sources of other beneficial nutrients, including vitamin C. Numerous studies show that, like beta-carotene, vitamin C offers protection against many cancers, including breast cancer.[1,2,10]

The debate over how much vitamin C humans require is ongoing. At one end of the spectrum, two-time Nobel Prize winner Linus Pauling and his followers recommend an intake somewhere between 2 and 9 grams a day during periods of health and even higher doses during times of stress or illness. At the other end of the spectrum, the Recommended Dietary Allowance (RDA) has been established at 60 milligrams for adults. Although I lean toward Pauling's recommendation (see Chapter 12), I want to stress that you should not rely on supplements to meet all your vitamin C requirements. Vitamin C–rich foods are rich in compounds, such as flavonoids and carotenes, that enhance the effects of vitamin C as well as exert favorable effects of their own.[11]

Most people think of citrus fruits as the best source of vitamin C. Vegetables also contain high levels—especially broccoli, peppers, potatoes, and Brussels sprouts. Vitamin C is destroyed by exposure to air. So, eating foods while they are as fresh as possible is the best way to get the most of their vitamin C. Although a salad from a salad bar is a healthful lunch choice, the vitamin C content of the fruits and vegetables is only a fraction of what it would be if the salad were made fresh. For example, freshly sliced cucumbers, if left standing, lose between 41% and 49% of their vitamin C content within the first three hours. A sliced cantaloupe, left uncovered in the refrigerator, loses 35% of its vitamin C in less than 24 hours.

Cabbage-Family Vegetables   The cabbage-family, or cruciferous vegetables, includes cabbage, broccoli, cauliflower, Brussels sprouts, kale, collard, mustard, radishes, rutabaga, turnips, and other common vegetables. One of the American Cancer Society's key dietary recommendations to reduce the risk of cancer is to include cruciferous vegetables in the diet.[17] Consumption of these foods has been shown to exert a protective effect against the development of many types of cancer, including breast cancer. The anticancer compounds in cabbage-family vegetables include phenols, indoles, isothiocyanates, and various sulfur-containing compounds. These compounds stimulate the body to detoxify and eliminate cancer-causing chemicals.

The anticancer effects of cabbage-family vegetables have been noted in numerous population studies.[1,2,10] Consistently, the higher the intake of cabbage-family vegetables, the lower the rates of cancer—particularly colon and breast cancer.[12-14] Broccoli is particularly beneficial. In addition to being especially rich in vitamin C and carotenes, compounds in broccoli (specifically, indole-3-carbinol) increase the excretion of the form of estrogen (2-hydroxyestrone) linked to breast cancer. Obviously, the regular consumption of broccoli and other cabbage-family vegetables is important in the battle against breast cancer.

Chapter 5 mentioned that cabbage-family vegetables contain goitrogens, compounds that can block the utilization of iodine. However, cooking inactivates goitrogens and there is no evidence that these compounds in cruciferous vegetables significantly interfere with thyroid function when dietary iodine is adequate. So, the presence of goitrogens in cruciferous vegetables should not worry you. Nonetheless, if you eat more than 4 servings per day of cruciferous vegetables, make sure your diet contains adequate iodine. Iodine is found in kelp and other seaweeds, vegetables grown near the sea, seafood, iodized salt, and in food supplements. Rutabagas and turnips contain the highest concentration of goitrogens.

The Importance of Fiber   Breast diseases, including fibrocystic breast disease (FBD) and breast cancer, have been linked to a low-fiber diet and bowel dysfunction. There is an interesting association between cellular abnormalities in breast fluid and the frequency of bowel movements.[18] Women having fewer than three bowel movements per week have a risk of FBD that is 4.5 times greater than that of women having at least one a day.

This association is probably due to the bacterial flora in the large intestine. These bacteria transform colon contents into a variety of toxic metabolites, including cancer-causing compounds.[19] Fecal microorganisms are capable of liberating estrogen from other compounds. Dietary fiber plays a major role in this regard. It influences the type of microflora present, the transit time of colon contents, the concentration of absorbable bowel toxins and metabolites, as well as the blood level of estrogens associated with breast cancer.[20,21]

Women on a vegetarian diet excrete two to three times more detoxified estrogens than women who eat meat.[6,22] Furthermore, meat-eating women have 50% higher mean levels of undetoxified estrogens in their blood. This evidence provides an additional reason for limiting the intake of animal products and increasing the consumption of plant foods.

Soy and Breast Cancer In June 1990, the National Cancer Institute held a workshop to examine the relationship between soybean consumption and cancer.[23,24] Soybean consumption is thought to be one of the major reasons for the relatively low rates of breast and colon cancers in Japan and China. Studies of animals have demonstrated that diets composed of as little as 5% soybeans can significantly inhibit chemically induced cancers. The most important anticancer compounds in soybeans, in relation to breast cancer, appear to be phytoestrogens (isoflavonoids and phytosterols).[6,20,21]

Garlic and Cancer The Greek physician Hippocrates prescribed eating garlic as treatment for cancers. Based on the results of modern animal research and some human studies, this recommendation was extremely wise. Several garlic components have displayed significant immune-enhancing as well as anticancer effects.[25] Human studies showing these effects are largely based on population studies. These studies reveal an inverse relationship between cancer rates and garlic consumption: Where cancer rates are lowest, garlic consumption is highest.

Garlic was somewhat effective at preventing mammary cancer in rats; when selenium-enriched garlic was used, an even greater effect was noted.[26] Selenium is an antioxidant mineral that functions very closely with vitamin E.

Perhaps the best (and most economical) way to get the benefits of garlic is to consume it regularly in the diet. A variety of commercial preparations on the market may also be of benefit. Simply follow the manufacturer's instructions.

Pesticides and Breast Cancer

The environment is contaminated with a group of compounds known as halogenated hydrocarbons. Included in this group are the toxic pesticides DDT, DDE, PCB, PCP, dieldrin, and chlordane. Pesticide residues may play a major role in breast cancer.

Molecules of halogenated hydrocarbons are hard to break down and are stored in fat cells. These chemicals are known to cause cancer in animals, but evidence for their causing cancer in humans is rare. These compounds have, however, been shown to suppress immune function, possess estrogenic activity, and alter hormone levels. All these effects could lead to breast cancer.

To evaluate the possible role of pesticides and pollutants in breast cancer, researchers measured the levels of these compounds in the fat cells of the breasts of women with malignant cancers and those with nonmalignant growths. The results? Higher levels of pesticide residues were found in the women with breast cancer. Although these results need to be confirmed, the association seems strong between pesticide levels in breast tissue and breast cancer.[27] This association is another compelling reason for choosing organically grown foods.

In the United States each year, over 1.2 billion pounds of pesticides and herbicides are sprayed on or added to crops. That is roughly 10 pounds of pesticides for each man, woman, and child. Although the pesticides are designed to affect insects and other organisms, experts estimate that only 2% of the pesticide actually serves its purpose. Over 98% is absorbed into the air, water, soil, or food supply. Most pesticides in use are synthetic chemicals of questionable safety. The major long-term health risks include the potential of causing cancer and birth defects. The major health risks of acute intoxication include vomiting, diarrhea, blurred vision, tremors, convulsions, and nerve damage.[28–30]

Because laboratory studies have not yet produced solid evidence that pesticide residues cause cancer in animals, many "experts" maintain that pesticides pose no significant risk for the public or the farmer. This opinion presents a major dilemma to scientists. What is more valid, studies of laboratory animals or population studies of humans? More and more evidence from human studies documents increased cancer and birth defect rates after pesticide exposure. This evidence indicates that pesticides are not as safe as the "experts" would like us to believe.

The history of pesticide use in this country is riddled with pesticides that were once widely used and then later banned due to health risks. Perhaps the best-known example is DDT. Used extensively from the early 1940s to 1973, DDT was largely responsible for increasing farm productivity in this country—but at what cost? DDT's hazards included infertility, birth defects, and other harmful effects. Unfortunately, although DDT has been banned for nearly 20 years, it is still found in the soil and in root vegetables such as carrots and potatoes. According to studies performed by the National Resources Defense Council, a public-interest environmental group, 17% of the carrots analyzed contained detectable levels of DDT.[31]

The majority of pesticides currently used in the United States are probably less toxic than DDT and other banned pesticides, such as Aldrin, dieldrin, endrin, and heptachlor. However, many pesticides banned in the United States are shipped to other countries, such as Mexico, which then send the food back to the United States. Although over 600 pesticides are currently used in the United States, most experts are most concerned about only a relative few. The Environmental Protection Agency has identified 64 pesticides as potential cancer-causing compounds; the National Research Council found that 80% of cancer risk due to pesticides is due to 13 pesticides used widely on 15 important food crops.[28] The pesticides are linuron, permethrin, chlordimeform, zineb, captafol, captan, maneb, mancozeb, folpet, chlorothalonil, metiram, benomyl, and O-phenylphenol. These pesticides are found in many crops, but residues are of greatest concern (in descending order) in tomatoes, beef, potatoes, oranges, lettuce, apples, peaches, pork, wheat, soybeans, beans, carrots, chicken, corn, and grapes.

State and federal regulatory agencies monitor pesticide residues and enforce legal tolerance levels. However, concern about the adequacy of the monitoring has been increasing. The EPA and FDA estimate that excessive pesticide residues are found on about 3% of domestic and 6% of foreign produce and that acceptable levels are found on 13% of domestic produce. Other organizations, however, report much higher levels. For example, the National Resources Defense Council conducted a survey of fresh produce sold in San Francisco markets. That group found that 44% of 71 fruits and vegetables had detectable levels of 19 different pesticides; 42% of produce with detectable pesticide residues contained more than one pesticide.[31] The sheer number and amount of pesticides showered on certain foods is astounding. For example, over 50 different pesticides are used on broccoli, 110 on apples, 70 on bell peppers, and so on.[28] Many of the pesticides penetrate the entire fruit or vegetable and cannot be washed off. Obviously, it is best to buy organic.

Many supermarket chains and produce suppliers are employing their own testing measures for determining the pesticide content of produce. Some are refusing to stock foods that have been treated with some of the more toxic pesticides, such as alachlor, captan, or EBDCs (ethylene bisdithiocarbamates). In addition, many stores are asking growers to disclose all pesticides used on foods and phase out the 64 pesticides suspected of causing cancers. Ultimately, it will be pressure from consumers that will have the greatest influence on food suppliers. Crop yield studies support the use of organic farming if the risk to human health is added to the equation.

How to Reduce Exposure to Pesticide Residues

The list that follows contains methods of reducing exposure to pesticides as well as tips on removing surface pesticide residues, waxes, fungicides, and fertilizers from produce.

1. Since pesticide residues are concentrated in animal fat, meat, eggs, cheese, and milk, avoid these foods.

2. Buy organic produce. In the context of food and farming, the term *organic* implies that the produce was grown without the aid of synthetic chemicals, including pesticides and fertilizers. In 1973, Oregon became the first state to pass laws that define criteria that produce must meet before it can be labeled as organic. By 1989, 16 other states (California, Colorado, Iowa, Maine, Massachusetts, Minnesota, Montana, Nebraska, New Hampshire, North Dakota, Ohio, South Dakota, Texas, Vermont, Washington, and Wisconsin) had adopted laws governing organic agriculture. Consumers should ask if produce is certified organic. If so, the next question should be By what organization is it certified? Highly reputable certification organizations include California Certified Organic Farmers, Demeter, Farm Verified Organic, Natural Organic Farmers Association, and the Organic Crop Improvement Association. Although less than 3% of the total produce grown in the United States is grown without the aid of pesticides, organic produce is widely available.

3. If organic produce is not readily available, develop a relationship with your local grocery-store produce manager. Explain to him or her your desire to reduce your exposure to pesticides and waxes. Ask what measures the store takes to ensure that pesticide residues are within the tolerance limits. Ask where the store gets its produce (foreign produce is much

more likely to contain excessive pesticides and banned pesticides than produce grown in the United States). Try to buy local produce that is in season.

4. To remove surface pesticide residues, waxes, fungicides, and fertilizers, soak the produce in a mild solution of additive-free soap, such as Ivory or pure castile soap from the health food store. You can also use an all-natural, biodegradable cleanser (available at most health food stores). Simply spray the produce with the cleanser, gently scrub, and then rinse. Or, simply peel off the skin or remove the outer layer of leaves. The downside of this is that many of the nutritional benefits are concentrated in the skin and outer layers.

The presence of pesticides in fruits and vegetables should not deter you from eating a diet rich in these foods. The concentrations in fruits and vegetables is much lower than the levels found in animal fats, meat, cheese, whole milk, and eggs. Furthermore, the various antioxidant components in fruits and vegetables help the body deal with the pesticides.

Final Comments

If you follow the dietary recommendations in this chapter and the guidelines in Chapter 11, your risk of breast cancer can be significantly reduced. If you have or have had breast cancer or if you are at high risk, follow these recommendations explicitly. They may greatly extend your life.

One additional recommendation: Avoid alcohol consumption. More than two dozen studies have clearly demonstrated that regular alcohol consumption increases the risk of breast cancer.[1] Although it is thought that consuming less than one drink per day is safe, drinking even a little more may increase the risk of breast cancer by as much as 50%.

9

Relief of Osteoarthritis

Postmenopausal women are at high risk for osteoarthritis and degenerative joint disease. Osteoarthritis is the most common form of arthritis and is seen primarily, but not exclusively, in the elderly. Surveys have indicated that over 40 million Americans have osteoarthritis, including 80% of persons over the age of 50. Under the age of 45, osteoarthritis is much more common in men; after age 45, it is 10 times more common in women than men.[1]

Osteoarthritis is the cumulative effect of decades of joint use. Long-term use stresses the integrity of the collagen matrix of cartilage. This cartilage damage results in the release of enzymes that destroy collagen components. With age, the ability to restore and manufacture normal collagen structures decreases.[1,2] The number as well as the activity of important repair enzymes is greatly reduced, making the joint structures especially prone to damage.

The weight-bearing joints (hips, spine, knees, and ankles) and joints of the hands are the joints most often affected by the degenerative changes associated with osteoarthritis.

Specifically, there is much cartilage destruction in joint margins. This is followed by hardening and the formation of large bone spurs. Pain, deformity, and limitation of motion in the joint results. Inflammation is usually minimal.[1]

The onset of osteoarthritis can be very subtle. Morning joint stiffness is often the first symptom. As the disease progresses, motion of the involved joint causes pain. Prolonged activity worsens the pain; pain is relieved by rest.

Aspirin and Other NSAIDs for Arthritis

The first drug generally used in the treatment of osteoarthritis and rheumatoid arthritis is aspirin. It is an example of a nonsteroidal anti-inflammatory drug, or NSAID. Other NSAIDs include fenoprofen (Nalfon), ibuprofen (Motrin, Advil, Nuprin), indomethacin (Indocin), naproxen (Naprosyn), piroxicam (Feldene), sulindac (Clinoril), and tolmetin (Tolectin).

Aspirin is often quite effective in relieving both the pain and inflammation. It is also relatively inexpensive. However, since the therapeutic dose required is relatively high (2 to 4 grams per day), toxicity often occurs. Tinnitus (ringing in the ears) and gastric irritation are early manifestations of toxicity.

Although other NSAIDS have not proven to be more effective than aspirin, some may be better tolerated. However, they are also much more expensive and present significant risk for side effects. Therefore, they are recommended for only short periods of time. In addition to being used for arthritis, NSAIDs are also used in the relief of headaches, low back pain, traumatic injury, postoperative pain, and menstrual cramps.

The specifics of how NSAIDs work have not been completely established. In general terms, however, they reduce inflammation by suppressing the formation of chemicals involved in the production of inflammation and pain. These chemicals are prostaglandins and related compounds.

Side Effects of NSAIDs

Since the dosage of NSAIDs necessary to suppress symptoms is usually quite high, so is the rate of side effects. The most common side effect of aspirin and other NSAIDs is damage to the intestinal tract and ulcer formation. In addition to causing ulcers, NSAIDs often cause allergic reactions, easy bleeding and bruising, ringing in the ears, and fluid retention. More serious complications include kidney and liver damage.

NSAIDs for Arthritis: More Harm Than Good?

One side effect of aspirin and other NSAIDs that is often not mentioned is inhibition of cartilage repair (that is, inhibition of collagen matrix synthesis) and acceleration of cartilage destruction.[3,4] Recall that osteoarthritis is caused by degeneration of cartilage. Although NSAIDs are fairly effective in suppressing osteoarthritis symptoms, they may worsen the condition by inhibiting cartilage formation and accelerating cartilage destruction.

In an effort to evaluate the effectiveness of current drug treatment of osteoarthritis, several studies attempted to determine the "natural course" of the disease.[3,5] In other words, these studies attempted to chart the course of the disease if no treatment was given. In one 10-year study of the natural course of osteoarthritis of the hip, all subjects initially had changes suggestive of advanced osteoarthritis. Yet the researchers reported remarkable clinical improvement, without therapy, in 14 of 31 hips at the end of the study.[5] X-ray films confirmed recovery of the joint space. In contrast, several studies have shown that NSAIDs accelerated osteoarthritis and increased joint destruction.[6-8] In other words, there is substantial evidence that people with osteoarthritis would be better off without NSAIDs.

Dietary Recommendations for Osteoarthritis

Perhaps the most important dietary recommendation for individuals suffering from osteoarthritis is to achieve normal body weight. Being overweight means increased stress on weight-bearing joints affected with osteoarthritis.

Both in terms of preventing and treating osteoarthritis with diet, it is critical to eat a diet rich in whole natural foods, especially raw fruits and vegetables. These foods supply nutrients critical to joint health, particularly antioxidant factors such as vitamin C, carotenes, and flavonoids. Especially beneficial are flavonoid-rich fruits such as cherries, blueberries, and blackberries. Also important are sulfur-containing foods such as garlic, onions, Brussels sprouts, and cabbage. The sulfur content of the fingernails of arthritis sufferers is lower than that of healthy people.[9] Normalizing the sulfur content of the nails was reported to alleviate pain and swelling of the joints, according to clinical data from the 1930s.[10] For some reason, this promising research was never pursued.

In the treatment of osteoarthritis, Norman Childers, Ph.D., popularized a diet that eliminated foods from the nightshade family. (He found that this simple dietary elimination cured his own osteoarthritis.)[11] Childers developed a theory that genetically susceptible individuals might develop arthritis, as well as a variety of other complaints, from long-term low-level consumption of the alkaloids found in tomatoes, potatoes, eggplant, peppers, and tobacco. Presumably, these alkaloids inhibit normal collagen repair in the joints or promote the inflammatory degeneration of the joint. To test his theory, Dr. Childers conducted an informal study of over 5,000 arthritis patients who agreed to avoid eating nightshade-family vegetables. Over 70% reported relief from aches and pains. Although remaining to be proved in a strict scientific study, the Childers diet may offer some benefit to certain individuals. It is certainly worth a try.

Glucosamine Sulfate

The general dietary recommendations given in this chapter are often quite effective on their own. There is much more that you can do about osteoarthritis and rheumatoid arthritis, however. Of particular importance is supplying adequate levels of antioxidant nutrients (such as selenium, manganese, and vitamins C and E) and those nutrients important in the manufacture of joint substances (especially niacinamide, pantothenic acid, vitamin B6, and zinc). Following the guidelines in Chapter 12 will provide ample levels of these key nutrients.

The single best natural treatment for osteoarthritis may be glucosamine sulfate. Glucosamine is a naturally occurring substance found in high concentrations in joint structures. The main function of glucosamine in joints is to stimulate the manufacture of the cartilage components necessary for joint repair. This action alone suggests a therapeutic role for glucosamine sulfate in osteoarthritis. But, there is much more. Glucosamine has also been shown to exert a protective effect against joint destruction and, when given orally as glucosamine sulfate, it is selectively taken up by joint tissues to exert a powerful therapeutic effect in osteoarthritis.

Numerous double-blind studies have shown that glucosamine sulfate produces much better results than NSAIDs and placebos in relieving the pain and inflammation of osteoarthritis.[12-15] NSAIDs offer purely symptomatic relief and may actually promote the disease process, but glucosamine sulfate addresses the cause of osteoarthritis. By getting at the root of the problem, glucosamine sulfate not only improves the symptoms, including pain, it also helps the body repair damaged joints. This is outstanding, but what is even more outstanding is the safety and the lack of side effects associated with oral glucosamine sulfate. In contrast, the side effects and risks associated with NSAIDs used in the treatment of osteoarthritis are significant. The therapeutic margin, a measure of safety, is 10 to 30 times more favorable for glucosamine sulfate than for commonly used NSAIDs, including aspirin.

The beneficial results of glucosamine are more obvious the longer it is used. Because glucosamine sulfate is not a pain-relieving substance per se, however, it does take a while to produce results. But, once it starts working, its results will outshine those of NSAIDs. For example, one study compared glucosamine sulfate to ibuprofen (Motrin). Pain scores decreased faster in the first two weeks in the ibuprofen group. However, by week 4, the group receiving the glucosamine sulfate was doing significantly better than the ibuprofen group.[11]

Glucosamine sulfate products are available at health food stores or through nutritionally oriented physicians. Be sure to use glucosamine sulfate, not glucosamine hydro-chloride or chlorhydrate, or *N*-acetyl-glucosamine. (The scientific studies that produced the best results used the sulfate form.) The standard dose for glucosamine sulfate is 500 milligrams, three times per day. As mentioned earlier, the human body tolerates glucosamine sulfate extremely well. In addition, there are no contraindications or adverse drug interactions. Glucosamine sulfate may cause some gastrointestinal upset (nausea, heartburn, and the like) in rare instances. If this occurs, try taking it during meals.

Glucosamine sulfate is a much better choice than chondroitin sulfate or cartilage preparations, including shark cartilage. Glucosamine is extremely effective when given orally; the effectiveness of oral chondroitin sulfate and cartilage products is a subject of considerable debate. Oral absorption studies of chondroitin sulfate estimate the absorption to be between 0% and 8%. Most of the studies of chondroitin sulfate that various manufacturers cite have utilized injectable forms. If chondroitin sulfate is effective orally, it is most likely because the body breaks it down into glucosamine.

Physical Therapy Modalities

Various physical therapy modalities (exercise, heat, cold, diathermy, ultrasound, and so on) performed by physical therapists, naturopathic physicians, and chiropractors are often very beneficial in improving joint mobility and reducing pain for sufferers of arthritis. The effect of physical therapy appears to be quite significant, especially when administered regularly by a trained professional.

10

Prevention of Heart Disease

The term *heart disease* is often used to describe disease of the blood vessels of the heart. These blood vessels are also called the coronary arteries. These arteries supply the heart muscle with vital oxygen and nutrients. If the blood flow through these arteries is restricted or blocked, severe damage or death to the heart muscle often occurs. This results in what is known as a heart attack. In most cases, the condition causing the blockage of blood and oxygen is atherosclerosis, or hardening of the artery walls due to a buildup of plaque. Plaque contains cholesterol, fatty material, and cellular debris.

Atherosclerosis and its complications are the major causes of death in the United States. In fact, more women than men die of heart disease. Heart disease accounts for 36% of all deaths in the United States. More than 52% of the fatalities caused by heart disease are women. Stroke, another complication of atherosclerosis, is the third most common cause of death in the United States. All together, atherosclerosis is responsible for at least 43% of all U.S.

deaths. The majority of these deaths involve postmenopausal women.

Atherosclerosis is largely a disease of diet and lifestyle;
therefore, many deaths due to heart disease could be significantly delayed by implementing a healthful diet and lifestyle.[1]

Cholesterol and Atherosclerosis

Foremost in the prevention and treatment of heart disease
is the reduction of blood cholesterol. The evidence overwhelmingly demonstrates that elevated cholesterol levels
greatly increase the risk of death due to heart disease.[1] The
first step in reducing the risk of heart disease is keeping
your total blood cholesterol level below 200 milligrams
per deciliter.

Not all cholesterol is bad; it serves many vital functions
in the body, including the manufacture of sex hormones
and bile acids. Without cholesterol many body processes
would not function properly. Cholesterol is transported in
the blood by molecules known as lipoproteins. Cholesterol
bound to low-density lipoprotein, or LDL, is often referred
to as "bad" cholesterol. Cholesterol bound to high-density
lipoprotein, or HDL, is often referred to as "good" cholesterol.
LDL cholesterol increases the risk of heart disease, stroke,
and high blood pressure. HDL cholesterol actually protects
against heart disease.[2]

LDL transports cholesterol to the tissues. HDL, on the
other hand, transports cholesterol to the liver, for metabolism and excretion from the body. Therefore, the HDL-to-
LDL ratio largely determines whether cholesterol is being
deposited into tissues or broken down and excreted. The
risk of heart disease can be reduced dramatically by lowering LDL cholesterol while raising HDL cholesterol. Research
has shown that, for every 1% drop in LDL cholesterol, the

Total cholesterol	Less than 200 mg/dL*
LDL cholesterol	Less than 130 mg/dL
HDL cholesterol	Greater than 35 mg/dL
Triglycerides	50–150 mg/dL

*milligrams per deciliter

Figure 10.1   Recommended blood cholesterol and triglyceride levels

risk of heart attack drops by 2%. Conversely, for every 1% increase in HDL, the risk of heart attack drops 3% to 4%.[2]

In addition to keeping an eye on your cholesterol level, it is also important to keep the level of triglycerides (other blood fats, or lipids, that increase the risk of heart disease) in the proper range. Figure 10.1 shows the recommended ranges for blood cholesterol and triglycerides.

Dietary Factors in Lowering Cholesterol

The most important approach to lowering a high cholesterol level is to follow a healthful diet. The dietary changes are simple: Eat less saturated fat and cholesterol by reducing or eliminating the amounts of animal products in the diet; increase the consumption of fiber-rich plant foods (fruits, vegetables, grains, and legumes); and lose weight, if necessary.

A number of medical organizations have developed specific guidelines for Americans to follow to reduce the risk of heart disease. Here are the key recommendations of the U.S. Surgeon General, the American Heart Association, and the National Research Council's Committee on Diet and Health:[1]

1. Reduce total fat intake to 30% or less of calories, reduce saturated fat intake to less than 10% of

calories, and reduce the intake of cholesterol to less than 300 milligrams daily.

2. Eat 5 or more servings of a combination of vegetables and fruits, especially green and yellow vegetables and citrus fruits.

3. Increase the intake of fiber and complex carbohydrates by eating 6 or more servings per day of a combination of breads, cereals, and legumes.

4. Maintain protein intake at moderate levels.

5. Balance food intake and physical activity to maintain appropriate body weight.

6. Limit the intake of alcohol, refined carbohydrates (sugar), and salt (sodium chloride).

Fish Oils

Since animal products are the primary sources of both saturated fats and cholesterol, it is obvious that the intake of animal products must be limited in order to prevent or reverse atherosclerosis. A possible exception to this recommendation about animal foods are cold-water fish. Salmon, mackerel, and herring provide oils known as omega-3 fatty acids. Hundreds of studies have shown that these beneficial oils lower cholesterol and triglyceride levels.[3,4]

The omega-3 fatty acids are not only being recommended to treat or prevent high cholesterol levels, but also high blood pressure; other cardiovascular diseases; cancer; autoimmune diseases, such as multiple sclerosis and rheumatoid arthritis; allergies and inflammation; eczema; psoriasis; and many others. Although the majority of studies of omega-3 oils have utilized fish oils (eicosapentaenoic acid [EPA] and docosahexaenoic acid [DHA]), flaxseed oil may offer similar benefit because it contains linolenic acid, an omega-3 oil that the body can convert to EPA. Linolenic acid exerts many of the same effects as EPA as well as several of its own.

A substantial body of evidence documents the beneficial effects of increasing the intake of fish oils in lowering blood cholesterol levels. The question remains, however: Should fish oils be taken as a supplement or should the dietary intake of fish be increased? In an effort to resolve this question, a recent five-week study of 25 men with high cholesterol levels compared the effects of eating fish oil from whole fish versus an equivalent amount of a fish oil supplement.[5] Although total cholesterol levels were unchanged in both groups, both fish and fish-oil supplements lowered triglycerides and raised HDL cholesterol.

Dietary fish did produce benefits that fish-oil supplements did not, however. Fish oils can reduce the "stickiness" of platelets and prevent clot formation. When platelets adhere to each other or aggregate to form a clot, this clot can get stuck in small arteries and produce a heart attack or stroke. In regard to reducing platelet stickiness, in this study dietary fish produced a much greater effect than fish-oil supplement. These findings suggest that, though both fish consumption and fish-oil supplementation produce desirable effects on lipids and lipoproteins, fish consumption is more effective in improving several other factors involved in cardiovascular disease.

If fresh cold-water fish are not readily available, I recommend supplementing the diet with either fish oils or flaxseed oil. The dosages found to be effective when using fish-oil supplements range from 5 to 15 grams of omega-3 fatty acids per day. Since most commercial products contain 500 milligrams of omega-3 fatty acids per capsule, this means a daily dose of 10 to 30 capsules. Although this can be expensive, it is much less expensive than cholesterol-lowering drugs, and it is certainly much safer. Flaxseed oil may indeed be the most advantageous oil for menopausal women, especially when cost-effectiveness is considered.

One tablespoon per day is all that is required. For best results, the flaxseed oil should definitely be cold-processed, to reduce rancidity. It can be used as a salad dressing or food supplement.

Nuts and Seeds

Another way of increasing the intake of health-promoting oils is to increase the consumption of nuts and seeds. As more Americans seek healthful food choices, nut and seed consumption is on the rise, and for good reason: Nuts and seeds are rich in many important nutrients, such as vitamin E, zinc, magnesium, and vitamin B6.

Because of the high oil content of nuts and seeds, you might suspect that the frequent consumption of nuts would increase the rate of obesity. But a study of 26,473 Americans found that the people who consumed the most nuts were the least obese.[6] A possible explanation is that the nuts produced satiety, a feeling of appetite satisfaction. The same study demonstrated that high nut consumption was associated with a protective effect against heart attacks (both fatal and nonfatal).

Nuts and seeds, due to their high oil content, are best purchased and stored in their shells. Make sure the shells are free from splits, cracks, stains, holes, or other surface imperfections. Do not eat or use moldy nuts or seeds— they can contain toxic substances. Also avoid limp, rubbery, dark, or shriveled nutmeats. Store nuts and seeds, in their shells, in a cool, dry environment. If whole nuts and seeds with their shells are unavailable, store the nutmeats in airtight containers in the refrigerator or freezer. Crushed, slivered, and nut pieces are the nut products most likely to be rancid. If a recipe calls for these, prepare your own from the whole nut.

Simple Food Substitutions

The importance of even simple alterations in diet can be quite significant. In one study, normal subjects ate two medium-sized carrots daily at breakfast.[7] After three weeks, the subjects' cholesterol level had dropped by 11%. Table 10.1 details some simple food choices that can lead to dramatic changes in your cholesterol levels and level of health.

Fiber-Rich Foods

Here is another example of how a simple food choice can affect cholesterol levels: Data from the National Health and Nutrition Examination Survey II (a national survey of the nutrition and health practices of Americans) disclosed that blood cholesterol levels are lowest among adults who eat whole-grain cereal for breakfast.[8] Although those individuals who consumed other breakfast foods had higher blood

Table 10.1 Food Choices for Lowering Cholesterol

Instead of These Foods	Eat These Foods
Red meats	Fish and white meat of poultry
Hamburgers and hot dogs	Soy-based alternatives
Eggs	Tofu, egg substitutes
High-fat dairy products	Lowfat or nonfat dairy products
Butter, lard, and other saturated fats	Vegetable oils
Ice cream, pies, cake, cookies, etc.	Fruits
Refined cereals, white bread, etc.	Whole grains, whole-wheat bread
Fried foods, fatty snack foods	Vegetables, fresh salads
Salt and salty foods	Low-sodium salt and low-salt foods
Coffee and soft drinks	Herbal teas, fresh fruit and vegetable juices

cholesterol levels, levels were highest among those who typically skipped breakfast.

Thanks to an explosion of marketing information, most Americans are aware of the cholesterol-lowering effects of oats. Since 1963, over 20 major clinical studies have examined the effect of oat bran on cholesterol levels.[9] Various oat preparations containing either oat bran or oatmeal have been studied, including cereals, muffins, breads, and entrées. The overwhelming majority of the studies demonstrated a very favorable effect on cholesterol levels. In individuals with high cholesterol levels (above 220 milligrams per deciliter), the consumption of the equivalent of 3 grams of water-soluble oat fiber typically lowers total cholesterol by 8% to 23%. This reduction is highly significant; as you have read, each 1% drop in total blood cholesterol means a 2% decrease in the risk of heart disease.

One bowl of ready-to-eat oat bran cereal or oatmeal provides about 3 grams of fiber. Although the fiber content of oatmeal (7%) is less than that of oat bran (15% to 26%), studies have determined that the polyunsaturated fatty acids in oatmeal contribute as much to the cholesterol-lowering effects of oats as the fiber content. Although oat bran has a higher fiber content, oatmeal is higher in polyunsaturated fatty acids. This makes oat bran and oatmeal equally effective. Although individuals with high cholesterol levels should see significant cholesterol reduction with frequent oat consumption, individuals with normal or low cholesterol levels will see little change.

A variety of other water-soluble fibers can lower cholesterol levels: psyllium, guar gum, and pectin. Eating a diet rich in whole grains, legumes (beans), and fresh fruit can provide high levels of these water-soluble fiber compounds. Although fiber supplements are becoming quite popular, it appears that eating foods rich in these water-soluble fibers makes more sense, from the health and financial perspectives.

To illustrate this, consider the effect of pectin, a remarkable type of fiber found in many fresh fruits, including pears, apples, grapefruit, and oranges. Pectin exerts a number of beneficial effects, including lowering cholesterol levels. In most of the studies of pectin and cholesterol, supplementing the diet with 15 grams of pectin produced a 10% drop in cholesterol levels.[10] Many people are buying high-priced drugs to get this kind of reduction. Since 15 grams of fiber is the amount of pectin in approximately 2 servings of fruit rich in pectin, eating 2 servings per day could lower the risk of heart disease by 20%. (Remember, for every 1% drop in total cholesterol, the risk of dying of a heart attack drops by 2%.) In addition to the pectin, these fruits would also provide important vitamins and minerals that can protect against heart disease.

Garlic and Onions

Garlic and onions exert numerous beneficial effects on the cardiovascular system. The benefits include lowering blood lipids and blood pressure. Numerous studies have demonstrated that both garlic and onions are effective in lowering LDL cholesterol and triglycerides while raising HDL cholesterol. In a 1979 population study, researchers studied three populations of vegetarians in the Jain community of India. Each population consumed a different amount of garlic and onions. As evident in Table 10.2, the most favorable effects were observed in the group that consumed the largest amount. The study is especially significant because the subjects had nearly identical diets, except in regard to garlic and onion ingestion.

Eating the equivalent of one clove of garlic or one-half onion per day will produce a 10% to 15% total reduction in total cholesterol in most people; others may require more. Although raw is best, even cooked garlic or onion produces some beneficial effects. You can also supplement your diet

Table 10.2 Effects of Garlic and Onion Consumption on Serum Lipids in Carefully Matched Diets

Garlic and Onion Consumption	Cholesterol	Triglycerides
Garlic 50 g/wk Onion 600 g/wk	159 mg/dL	52 mg/dL
Garlic 10 g/wk Onion 200 g/wk	172 mg/dL	75 mg/dL
No garlic or onions	208 mg/dL	109 mg/dL

by using one of the wide variety of different forms of garlic that exist on the marketplace, including so-called deodorized garlic. Use well-respected brands available at health food stores.

Lifestyle Factors in Lowering Cholesterol

Quit smoking! Statistical evidence reveals that smokers' risk of heart disease is three to five times that of nonsmokers. The more cigarettes smoked and the longer the period as a smoker, the greater the risk of dying from a heart attack or stroke.

Exercise! Many studies have shown a direct relationship between physical activity and cholesterol levels. Physical exercise is also associated with a decreased risk of heart disease and stroke.

Reduce or eliminate your consumption of coffee, both caffeinated and decaffeinated.

The Reversal of Heart Disease

More and more evidence is accumulating that the right diet and lifestyle are not only effective in preventing heart disease, but can also dramatically contribute to unclogging arteries. This reversal is perhaps best illustrated in the now-famous Lifestyle Heart Trial conducted by Dr. Dean Ornish.[11] In this study, subjects with heart disease were divided into a control group and an experimental group. The control group received regular medical care while the experimental group ate a lowfat vegetarian diet for at least one year. The diet included fruits, vegetables, grains, legumes, and soybean products. Subjects on the diet were allowed to consume as many calories as they wished. No animal products were allowed except egg white and 1 cup per day of nonfat milk or yogurt. The diet contained approximately 10% fat; 15% to 20% protein; and 70% to 75% carbohydrate, which was predominantly complex carbohydrate from whole grains, legumes, and vegetables.

The experimental group practiced stress reduction—such as breathing and stretching exercises, meditation, imagery, and other relaxation techniques—for an hour each day. In addition, these subjects exercised at least 3 hours a week. At the end of the year, the subjects in the experimental group showed significant overall regression of atherosclerosis of the coronary blood vessels. In contrast, subjects in the control group, who were being treated with regular medical care and following the standard American Heart Association diet, actually showed progression of their disease. In other words, the control group actually got worse. Ornish states: "This finding suggests that conventional recommendations for patients with coronary heart disease (such as a 30% fat diet) are not sufficient to bring about regression in many patients."

Although most authorities now agree that the level of blood cholesterol is largely determined by the dietary intake of total calories of cholesterol, saturated fat, and polyunsaturated fat, the result of Ornish's study and other studies suggests that other factors are also important.

Strict vegetarianism may not be as important as consuming a diet high in fiber and complex carbohydrates, low in fat, and low in cholesterol. It is well established, however, that vegetarians have a much lower risk of developing heart disease and that a vegetarian diet is quite effective in lowering cholesterol levels and reducing the risk of atherosclerosis.[12]

By following the dietary recommendations given in Chapter 11, you will ensure that your diet is rich in factors that protect against heart disease. These include fiber, essential fatty acids, vitamins, potassium, and magnesium.

Inositol Hexaniacinate

If additional means of lowering cholesterol are required, inositol hexaniacinate (a safe form of niacin) is recommended. Niacin has long been used to lower cholesterol levels. In fact, niacin is recommended by the National Cholesterol Education Program as the first "drug" to use.[13] Niacin was the only substance to demonstrate a decreased mortality in the famed Coronary Drug Project.[14] The problem with niacin is that the dose required (1 gram, three times per day) often results in flushing of the skin, stomach irritation, ulcers, liver damage, fatigue, and other side effects. Because of these side effects, it is often recommended that niacin therapy for lowering cholesterol be supervised by a physician.

Inositol hexaniacinate is composed of one molecule of inositol (an unofficial B vitamin) and six molecules of niacin. Inositol hexaniacinate has been used in Europe for over 30 years to lower cholesterol levels and also to improve blood flow. It yields slightly better results than standard niacin, and the body tolerates it better. Compared to niacin, inositol hexaniacinate causes less flushing and fewer long-term side effects, including effects on blood sugar control.[15–17] Inositol hexaniacinate is available at health food stores. The best dosage for lowering cholesterol levels is 1,000 to 3,000 milligrams per day.

III

Beyond Menopause

The chapters in this section provide a foundation for good health well beyond menopause. Achieving and maintaining health is usually quite easy if you implement a few basic principles: Maintain a positive mental attitude, follow a healthful diet, and exercise. In addition, modern life seems to make supplementing the diet with essential nutrients necessary.

Ralph Waldo Emerson said, "The first wealth is health." Nevertheless, trying to sell people on health is often difficult. To be healthy takes commitment. The reward is not always readily seen or felt. It is usually not until the body fails us in some manner that we realize that we haven't taken care of it.

The reward for most people who maintain a positive mental attitude, eat a healthful diet, exercise regularly, and supplement their diet with essential nutrients is a life filled with very high levels of vitality and a tremendous passion for living.

11

Dietary Guidelines

There is an ever-growing appreciation of the role of diet in determining the level of health. In fact, it is now well established that dietary practices cause, as well as prevent, a wide range of diseases. In addition, an accumulation of research indicates that certain diets and foods offer immediate therapeutic benefit.

There is little debate that a healthful diet must be rich in whole "natural" and unprocessed foods. Of particular importance are plant foods, such as fruits, vegetables, grains, beans, seeds, and nuts. These foods contain not only valuable nutrients, but also dietary fiber and other food compounds that have remarkable health-promoting properties. A diet rich in plant foods offers significant protection against the development of chronic degenerative problems, such as heart disease, cancer, diabetes, stroke, and arthritis.[1-3] Figure 11.1 lists diseases associated with a diet low in plant foods.

Metabolic diseases: Obesity, diabetes, kidney stones, gallstones, gout

Cardiovascular diseases: Hypertension, cerebrovascular disease, ischemic heart disease, varicose veins, deep vein thrombosis, pulmonary embolism

Gastrointestinal diseases: Constipation, appendicitis, diverticulitis, diverticulosis, hemorrhoids, colon cancer, irritable bowel syndrome, ulcerative colitis, Crohn's disease

Other diseases: Dental caries, autoimmune disorders (including multiple sclerosis), thyrotoxicosis, many skin conditions

Figure 11.1   Diseases associated with a diet low in plant foods

The Government and Nutrition Education

Throughout the years various government organizations have published dietary guidelines, but it has been the recommendations of the United States Department of Agriculture (USDA) that have become the most widely known. In 1956, the USDA published "Food for Fitness—A Daily Food Guide." This guide categorized food into the Basic Four Food Groups. The Basic Four consisted of:

1. The Milk Group: Milk, cheese, ice cream, and other milk-based foods
2. The Meat Group: Meat, fish, poultry, and eggs, with dried legumes and nuts as alternatives
3. The Fruit and Vegetable Group
4. The Breads and Cereals Group

One of the major problems with the Basic Four Food Groups model is that it graphically suggests that the food groups are equal in health value. The result: overconsumption of animal products, dietary fat, and refined carbohydrates, and insufficient consumption of fiber-rich foods such as fruits, vegetables, and legumes. Following such a diet has resulted in many premature deaths, chronic diseases, and

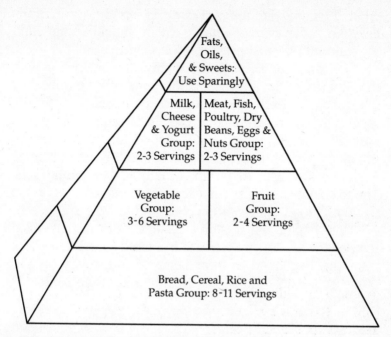

Figure 11.2 The eating right food pyramid

increased health care costs. According to the U.S. Surgeon General's Report on Nutrition and Health, diet-related diseases account for 68% of all deaths in this country.[2]

In an attempt to create a new model in nutrition education, the USDA developed the Eating Right Pyramid. This model does not change the food groups per se. Instead, it visually stresses the importance of making fresh fruits, vegetables, and whole grains the basis of a healthful diet. Figure 11.2 presents the Eating Right Pyramid.

The Design of a Healthful Diet

Most people give very little thought to the design of their diet. They are motivated to eat by sensual needs rather than what their body requires. Health is largely a conscious decision. Awareness of what to eat, in what quantities, and of healthful ways to prepare food is critical.

The American Dietetic Association, in conjunction with the American Diabetes Association and other groups, has developed the Exchange System, a convenient tool for the rapid estimation of the calorie, protein, fat, and carbohydrate content of a diet. Originally intended for use in designing dietary recommendations for diabetics, the Exchange System is now used to design virtually all therapeutic diets. The Exchange System does not place enough stress on the quality of food choices, however.

This chapter will present a system of diet design called the Healthy Exchange System. It is a more beneficial system than the Exchange System because it focuses on unprocessed, whole foods. The Healthy Exchange System is based on seven lists:

List 1	Vegetables
List 2	Fruits
List 3	Breads, cereals, and starchy vegetables
List 4	Legumes
List 5	Fats and oils
List 6	Milk
List 7	Meats, fish, cheese, and eggs

Lists 6 and 7—the milk and meat lists—are optional. All food portions within each list provide approximately the same calories, proteins, fats, and carbohydrates. (The fact that the servings are equal in this sense gives rise to the term *exchange*—for the most part, any item in one list can be exchanged for any item in the same list.)

To use the Healthy Exchange System, you begin by determining your body frame size. Knowing this allows you to calculate the number of calories you need each day to maintain yourself healthfully. Then you turn to the diets of the Healthy Exchange System. These are "menus" that tell you how many servings from each Healthy Exchange List you should eat to consume the number of calories appropriate for you. You must then decide whether you will be a vegan (someone who does not consume meat or dairy products) or an omnivore (someone who eats animal and vegetable substances). At each specific calorie level, the Healthy Exchange System offers a vegan and an omnivore diet. Later in this chapter, you will determine your frame size, calculate the number of daily calories you need, and examine each Exchange List in detail.

Because all food portions within each Exchange List provide approximately the same calories, proteins, fats, and carbohydrates per serving, it is easy to construct a diet that has the following components:

Carbohydrates	65% to 75% of total calories
Fats	15% to 25% of total calories
Protein	10% to 15% of total calories
Dietary fiber	At least 50 grams

Of the carbohydrates ingested, 90% should be complex carbohydrates or naturally occurring sugars. Limit intake of refined carbohydrates and concentrated sugars (including honey, pasteurized fruit juices, and dried fruit, as well as sugar and white flour) to less than 10% of the total calorie intake. Table 11.1 shows the fat, carbohydrate, and protein composition per serving for each Exchange List.

How Many Calories Do You Need?

The first step in determining your caloric needs is to determine the size of your body frame. The next step is to determine ideal body weight and calculate the number of calories necessary to sustain that weight.

Table 11.1   Macronutrient Composition Per Serving

Healthy Exchange System List	Protein (g)	Fat (g)	Carbo-hydrates (g)	Fiber (g)	Calories (kcal)
Vegetables	3.0	0.0	11.0	1.0–3.0	50
Fruits	0.0	0.0	20.0	1.0–3.0	80
Breads, etc.	2.0	0.0	15.0	1.0–4.0	70
Legumes	7.0	0.5	15.0	6.0–7.0	90
Fats and oils	0.0	5.0	0.0	0.0	45
Milk	8.0	0.0	12.0	0.0	80
Meats, etc.	7.0	3.0	0.0	0.0	55

Determining Frame Size   Extend your arm and bend the forearm upward at a 90-degree angle. Keep the fingers straight and turn the inside of your wrist away from your body. Place the thumb and index finger of your other hand on the two prominent bones on either side of your elbow. Measure the space between your fingers with a tape measure. Table 11.2 presents data for men and women; choose the data appropriate for you. Find your height in the left column. Compare the measurement of the breadth of your elbow with the elbow measurement beside your height. The elbow measurements are for medium-framed individuals. If the breadth of your elbow is smaller than the range cited in the table, you have a small frame; if it is larger, you have a large frame.

Now that you know the size of your body frame, you can determine the body weight appropriate for it.

Determining Ideal Body Weight   The most popular tables of "desirable" weight are those provided by the Metropolitan Life Insurance Company. The most recent edition of these

Table 11.2 Data for the Calculation of Body Frame Size

Height in 1″ Heels	Elbow Breadth
Men	
5′2″–5′3″	2½–2⅞″
5′4″–5′7″	2⅝–2⅞″
5′8″–5′11″	2¾–3″
6′0″–6′3″	2¾–3⅛″
6′4″	2⅞–3¼″
Women	
4′10″–5′3″	2¼–2½″
5′4″–5′11″	2⅜–2⅝″
6′0″	2½–2¾″

tables, published in 1983, gives weight ranges for men and women, in 1-inch increments of height, for three body frame sizes. Table 11.3 presents the Metropolitan Life Insurance tables of desirable weight.

The next step in determining your daily caloric needs is to make a calculation involving weight and activity level.

Factoring In Your Activity Level Convert your ideal weight in pounds to kilograms by multiplying it by 0.4536. Next choose, from the list that follows, the activity level that best describes you.

Little physical activity	30 calories
Light physical activity	35 calories
Moderate physical activity	40 calories
Heavy physical activity	45 calories

Make a note of the number of calories cited for the level you chose. You will use this number in the equation that

Table 11.3   1983 Metropolitan Life Insurance Tables of Ideal
Body Weight*

Height	Small Frame	Weight (lb) Medium Frame	Large Frame
Men			
5'2"	128–134	131–141	138–150
5'3"	130–136	133–143	140–153
5'4"	132–138	135–145	142–156
5'5"	134–140	137–148	144–160
5'6"	136–142	139–151	146–164
5'7"	138–145	142–154	149–168
5'8"	140–148	145–157	152–172
5'9"	142–151	148–160	155–176
5'10"	144–154	151–163	158–180
5'11"	146–157	154–166	161–184
6'0"	149–160	157–170	164–188
6'1"	152–164	160–174	168–192
6'2"	155–168	164–178	172–197
6'3"	158–172	167–182	176–202
6'4"	162–176	171–187	181–207
Women			
4'10"	102–111	109–121	118–131
4'11"	103–113	111–123	120–134
5'0"	104–115	113–126	122–137
5'1"	106–118	115–129	125–140
5'2"	108–121	118–132	128–143
5'3"	111–124	121–135	131–147
5'4"	114–127	124–138	134–151
5'5"	117–130	127–141	137–155
5'6"	120–133	130–144	140–159
5'7"	123–136	133–147	143–163
5'8"	126–139	136–150	146–167
5'9"	129–142	139–153	149–170
5'10"	132–145	142–156	152–173
5'11"	135–148	145–159	155–176
6'0"	138–151	148–162	158–179

*Weights cited are, in pounds, for adults age 25–59, based on lowest
mortality. Weight is cited according to frame size in indoor clothing
(5 pounds for men and 3 pounds for women), wearing shoes with 1" heels.

calculates the number of calories you need each day. The equation follows.

		Number of calories for		Approximate daily calorie
Weight (in kg)	×	activity level	=	requirements
____	×	____	=	____ calories

For example, I weigh 195 pounds. That amount multiplied by 0.4536 equals 88.452, or about 88 kilograms. I would rate my physical activity level as moderate. (Even though I exercise at least 5 days a week for a minimum of 1 hour, during most of the day I am sedentary.) Therefore, the equation to calculate my daily caloric needs looks like this:

$$88 \times 40 = 3{,}520 \text{ calories}$$

Now that you know your daily caloric needs, you are ready to take a look at the diets of the Healthy Exchange System.

The Diets of the Healthy Exchange System

As you recall, the Healthy Exchange System defines seven lists—five mandatory and two optional—that categorize foods according to broad groups. The diets of the Healthy Exchange System define the number of servings you should eat from each list. The diets provide total daily calories in the range of 1,000 to 3,000 calories, in increments of 500 calories. The system offers two diets at each level: one for the vegan and one for the omnivore.

As an example of one of the diets, study the 1,500-calorie vegan diet, which follows.

1,500-Calorie Vegan Diet (daily intake)

List 1 (vegetables)	5 servings
List 2 (fruits)	2 servings

List 3 (breads, cereals, and starchy vegetables)   9 servings

List 4 (legumes)   2.5 servings

List 5 (fats and oils)   4 servings

This diet results in an intake of approximately 1,500 calories, of which 67% is derived from complex carbohydrates and naturally occurring sugars, 18% from fats, and 15% from proteins. The protein intake is entirely from plant sources, but still provides approximately 55 grams of protein, an amount well above the recommended daily allowance, or RDA, for someone requiring 1,500 calories. At least one-half of the fat servings should be from nuts, seeds, and other whole foods from list 5, the fat exchange list. The dietary fiber intake is 31 to 74.5 grams. The list that follows summarizes this information.

Percentage of calories as carbohydrates: 67%

Percentage of calories as fats: 18%

Percentage of calories as protein: 15%

Protein content: 55 grams

Dietary fiber content: 31 to 74.5 grams

The remainder of this section presents the other diets of the Healthy Exchange System. Find the one that is right for you.

1,500-Calorie Omnivore Diet (daily intake)

List 1 (vegetables)   5 servings

List 2 (fruits)   2.5 servings

List 3 (breads, cereals, and starchy vegetables)   6 servings

List 4 (legumes)   1 serving

List 5 (fats and oils)   5 servings

List 6 (milk)   1 serving
List 7 (meats, fish, cheese, and eggs)   2 servings
   Percentage of calories as carbohydrates: 67%
   Percentage of calories as fats: 18%
   Percentage of calories as protein: 15%
   Protein content: 61 grams (75% from plant sources)
   Dietary fiber content: 19.5 to 53.5 grams

2,000-Calorie Vegan Diet (daily intake)
List 1 (vegetables)   5.5 servings
List 2 (fruits)   2 servings
List 3 (breads, cereals, and starchy   11 servings
vegetables)
List 4 (legumes)   5 servings
List 5 (fats and oils)   8 servings
   Percentage of calories as carbohydrates: 67%
   Percentage of calories as fats: 18%
   Percentage of calories as protein: 15%
   Protein content: 79 grams
   Dietary fiber content: 48.5 to 101.5 grams

2,000-Calorie Omnivore Diet (daily intake)
List 1 (vegetables)   5 servings
List 2 (fruits)   2.5 servings
List 3 (breads, cereals, and starchy   13 servings
vegetables)
List 4 (legumes)   2 servings
List 5 (fats and oils)   7 servings
List 6 (milk)   1 serving
List 7 (meats, fish, cheese, and eggs)   2 servings
   Percentage of calories as carbohydrates: 66%
   Percentage of calories as fats: 19%

Percentage of calories as protein: 15%
Protein content: 78 grams (72% from plant sources)
Dietary fiber content: 32.5 to 88.5 grams

2,500-Calorie Vegan Diet (daily intake)

List 1 (vegetables)	8 servings
List 2 (fruits)	3 servings
List 3 (breads, cereals, and starchy vegetables)	17 servings
List 4 (legumes)	5 servings
List 5 (fats and oils)	8 servings

Percentage of calories as carbohydrates: 69%
Percentage of calories as fats: 15%
Percentage of calories as protein: 16%
Protein content: 101 grams
Dietary fiber content: 33 to 121 grams

2,500-Calorie Omnivore Diet (daily intake)

List 1 (vegetables)	8 servings
List 2 (fruits)	3.5 servings
List 3 (breads, cereals, and starchy vegetables)	17 servings
List 4 (legumes)	2 servings
List 5 (fats and oils)	8 servings
List 6 (milk)	1 serving
List 7 (meats, fish, cheese, and eggs)	3 servings

Percentage of calories as carbohydrates: 66%
Percentage of calories as fats: 18%
Percentage of calories as protein: 16%
Protein content: 102 grams (80% from plant sources)
Dietary fiber content: 40.5 to 116.5 grams

3,000-Calorie Vegan Diet (daily intake)

List 1 (vegetables)	10 servings
List 2 (fruits)	4 servings
List 3 (breads, cereals, and starchy vegetables)	17 servings
List 4 (legumes)	6 servings
List 5 (fats and oils)	10 servings

Percentage of calories as carbohydrates: 70%

Percentage of calories as fats: 16%

Percentage of calories as protein: 14%

Protein content: 116 grams

Dietary fiber content: 50–84 grams

3,000-Calorie Omnivore Diet (daily intake)

List 1 (vegetables)	10 servings
List 2 (fruits)	3 servings
List 3 (breads, cereals, and starchy vegetables)	20 servings
List 4 (legumes)	2 servings
List 5 (fats and oils)	10 servings
List 6 (milk)	1 serving
List 7 (meats, fish, cheese, and eggs)	3 servings

Percentage of calories as carbohydrates: 67%

Percentage of calories as fats: 18%

Percentage of calories as protein: 15%

Protein content: 116 grams (81% from plant sources)

Dietary fiber content: 45 to 133 grams

Note: Use these diets as the basis for calculating diets of specific calorie amounts. For example, for a 4,000-calorie diet, add the 2,500-calorie diet to the 1,500-calorie diet. For a 1,000-calorie diet, divide the 2,000-calorie diet in half.

In the next seven sections you will examine each exchange list in the Healthy Exchange System. You will learn about the general characteristics of each category of food and how individual foods can benefit you or be detrimental to nutrition. In each section, an exchange list appears. From these lists, each day, you will choose foods to meet the serving requirements defined by your diet.

List 1: Vegetables

Vegetables provide the broadest range of nutrients of any food class. They are rich sources of vitamins, minerals, carbohydrates, and proteins. The little fat they contain is in the form of essential fatty acids. In addition, vegetables provide high quantities of other valuable health-promoting substances, especially carotenes (substances that can be converted into vitamin A) and fiber. In Latin, the word *vegetable* means to enliven or animate. Vegetables give us life. More and more evidence is accumulating that shows that vegetables can prevent as well as treat many diseases.

Vegetables should play a major role in the diet. The U.S. National Academy of Science, the U.S. Department of Health and Human Services, and the National Cancer Institute recommend that Americans consume a minimum of 3 to 5 servings of vegetables per day.[2] I recommend 8 servings per day.

The best way to consume many vegetables is in their fresh, raw form. In this form, many of their nutrients and health-promoting compounds are provided in much higher concentrations than in processed vegetables. Drinking fresh vegetable juice is an excellent way to make sure you are achieving your daily quota of vegetables.

When cooking vegetables, be sure not to overcook them. Overcooking will not only result in the loss of important nutrients, it will alter the flavor. Light steaming, baking, and quick stir-frying are the best ways to cook vegetables. Do not boil vegetables; most of the nutrients will be left in the water. The only exception to this rule is soup making. Since the liquid used for boiling the vegetables is the soup itself, and you will consume the soup, boiling soup vegetables is fine. If, for soup or other dishes, fresh vegetables are not available, frozen vegetables are preferred over their canned counterparts.

Although pickled vegetables are quite popular, they may not be healthful choices. Not only are they high in salt, they may also be high in cancer-causing compounds. Several population studies in China have suggested an association between consumption of pickled vegetables and cancer of the esophagus.[4] Pickled vegetables contain high concentrations of *N*-nitroso compounds. Once ingested, these compounds can form potent cancer-causing nitrosamines.

Vegetables are fantastic "diet" foods because they are very high in nutritional value but low in calories. In list 1 you will notice a category for "free" vegetables. These vegetables are termed free because you can eat them in any amount desired; the calories they contain will be offset by the number of calories your body will burn to digest them. If you are trying to lose weight, these foods are especially valuable because they will help to keep you feeling satisfied between meals.

Vegetables

Measured-serving vegetables

Unless otherwise noted, 1 serving consists of 1 cup of cooked vegetables or fresh vegetable juice or 2 cups of raw vegetable.

Artichoke (1 medium)
Asparagus
Bean sprouts
Beets

Broccoli
Brussels sprouts
Carrots
Cauliflower
Eggplant
Greens
    Beet
    Chard
    Collard
    Dandelion
    Kale
    Mustard
    Spinach (cooked)
    Turnip
Mushrooms
Okra
Onions
Rhubarb
Rutabaga
Sauerkraut
String beans, green or yellow
Summer squash
Tomatoes, tomato juice, vegetable juice cocktail
Zucchini

Free vegetables
Eat as many of the following items as you wish.
Alfalfa sprouts
Bell peppers
Bok choy
Cabbage

Celery
Chicory
Chinese cabbage
Cucumber
Endive
Escarole
Lettuce
Parsley
Radishes
Spinach (raw)
Turnips
Watercress

List 2: Fruits

Fruits are excellent sources of many vital antioxidants, such as vitamin C, carotenes, and flavonoids. However, fruits are not as dense in nutrients as vegetables, because they tend to be higher in calories. That is why vegetables are favored over fruits. Nonetheless, regular fruit consumption has been shown to offer significant protection against many chronic degenerative diseases, including cancer, heart disease, cataracts, and stroke.[3]

Since fruits contain a fair amount of natural fruit sugar, or fructose, most responsible eating programs recommend limiting your intake to no more than 4 servings of fruit or two 8-ounce glasses of fresh fruit juice per day. Fruits make excellent snacks because fructose is absorbed slowly into the bloodstream, thereby allowing the body time to utilize it.

The Healthy Exchange List for fruit follows. You will note that the list includes a few items made from processed fruit—jams, jellies, and preserves—and a few items that are not fruits at all—honey and sugar. Do not eat more than 1 serving per day of these processed products.

Fruits

Each of the following items equals 1 serving.

Fresh fruit and fruit-based items
Fresh juice, 1 cup (8 ounces)*
Pasteurized juice, ⅔ cup

Apple, 1 large
Applesauce (unsweetened), 1 cup
Apricots, dried, 8 halves
Apricots, fresh, 4 medium
Banana, 1 medium
Berries
    Blackberries, 1 cup
    Blueberries, 1 cup
    Cranberries, 1 cup
    Raspberries, 1 cup
    Strawberries, 1½ cups
Cherries, 20 large
Dates, 4
Figs, dried, 2
Figs, fresh, 2
Grapefruit, 1
Grapefruit juice, 1 cup
Grapes, 20
Mango, 1 small
Melons
    Cantaloupe, ½ small
    Honeydew, ¼ medium
    Watermelon, 2 cups
Nectarines, 2 small
Orange, 1 large

Papaya, 1½ cups

Peach, 2 medium

Persimmon, native, 2 medium

Pineapple, 1 cup

Plums, 4 medium

Prune juice, ½ cup

Prunes, 4 medium

Raisins, 4 tablespoons

Tangerines, 2 medium

Processed fruit and other products

Eat no more than 1 serving of the following "fruit" foods per day.

Honey, 1 tablespoon

Jams, jellies, preserves, 1 tablespoon

Sugar, 1 tablespoon

*Although 1 cup of most fruit juices equals 1 serving, prune juice is an exception; consult the alphabetized portion of the list.

List 3: Breads, Cereals, and Starchy Vegetables

Breads, cereals, and starchy vegetables are classified as complex carbohydrates. Complex carbohydrates are made up of long chains of simple carbohydrates, or sugars. This means the human body has to digest, or break down, the large sugar chains into simple sugars. Therefore, the sugar from complex carbohydrates enters the bloodstream slowly. This means a relatively stable blood sugar level and appetite.

Complex carbohydrates—breads, cereals, and starchy vegetables—are higher in fiber and nutrients and lower in calories than simple-sugar items such as cakes and candies.

Choose whole-grain products (whole-grain breads, whole-grain flour products, brown rice, and the like) over their processed counterparts (white bread, white-flour products, white rice, and so on). Whole grains are a major source of complex carbohydrates, dietary fiber, minerals, and B vitamins. The protein content and quality of whole grains is greater than that of refined grains. Diets rich in whole grains guard against chronic degenerative diseases. Whole-grain foods are especially significant in the prevention of breast cancer, heart disease, diabetes, varicose veins, and diseases of the colon (such as colon cancer, inflammatory bowel disease, hemorrhoids, and diverticulitis).[2]

Whole grains can be used as breakfast cereals, side dishes, or casseroles or as part of a dinner entrée. Whole-grain recipes appear later in this chapter. Another of my books, *The Healing Power of Foods Cookbook* (Prima Publishing, Rocklin, CA, 1993) also contains many whole-grain recipes.

Note that some of the prepared foods included in the list of breads, cereals, and starchy vegetables constitute more than 1 serving.

Breads, Cereals, and Starchy Vegetables
Each of the following items equals 1 serving.
    Breads
            Bagel, small, ½
            Dinner roll, 1
            Dried bread crumbs, 3 tablespoons
            English muffin, small, ½
            Tortilla (6 inch), 1
            Whole wheat, rye, or pumpernickel, 1 slice
    Cereals
            Bran flakes, ½ cup
            Cornmeal (dry), 2 tablespoons

Flour, 2½ tablespoons
Grits (cooked), ½ cup
Pasta (cooked), ½ cup
Porridge (cooked cereal), ½ cup
Puffed cereal (unsweetened), 1 cup
Rice or barley (cooked), ½ cup
Unpuffed unsweetened cereal, ¾ cup
Wheat germ, ¼ cup

Crackers
Arrowroot, 3
Graham (2½-inch squares), 2
Matzo (4 by 6 inches), ½
Rye wafers (2 by 3½ inches), 3
Saltine, 6

Starchy vegetables
Corn, kernels, ⅓ cup
Corn on the cob, 1 small cob
Parsnips, ⅔ cup
Potato, mashed, ½ cup
Potato, white, 1 small
Squash (acorn, butternut, or winter), ½ cup
Yam or sweet potato, ¼ cup

Prepared foods

Each of the following items equals 1 "bread" serving, but you must omit 1 or more fat servings to maintain the nutrition balance of your diet.

Biscuit, 2-inch diameter, 1 (omit 1 fat serving)
Corn bread, 2 by 2 by 1 inch, 1 (omit 1 fat serving)
French fries, 2 to 3 inches long, 8 (omit 1 fat serving)
Muffin, small, 1 (omit 1 fat serving)
Pancake, 5 by ½ inch, 1 (omit 1 fat serving)

Potato or corn chips, 15 (omit 2 fat servings)
Waffle, 5 by ½ inch, 1 (omit 1 fat serving)

List 4: Legumes

According to the dictionary, a legume is a plant that produces a pod that splits on both sides. Of the common human foods, beans, peas, lentils, and peanuts are legumes. The legume category also includes alfalfa, clover, acacia, and indigo. The fossil record indicates that legumes are among the oldest cultivated plants; prehistoric peoples domesticated and cultivated certain legumes for food. Today, legumes are a mainstay in most diets of the world. Legumes are second only to grains in supplying calories and protein to the human population. Compared to grains, they supply about the same number of total calories, but usually provide two to four times as much protein.

Legumes are often called the poor people's meat; however, they might be better known as the healthy people's meat. Although lacking some key amino acids, legumes can be combined with grains to form what is known as a complete protein. Many legumes, especially soybeans, provide impressive health benefits. Diets rich in legumes are being used to lower cholesterol levels, improve blood glucose control in diabetics, and reduce the risk of many cancers. Obviously, legumes are an important part of a healthful diet.

This book has stressed the benefits of legumes, particularly soy. In addition to the phytoestrogen action, the phytosterols of legumes, as well as most nuts and seeds, also exert well-documented cholesterol-lowering effects.[5] Phytosterols can enhance immune function, inhibit the Epstein-Barr virus, prevent chemically induced cancers in animals, and exhibit numerous anticancer effects.[6] Some researchers think the body may be able to utilize phytosterols in hormone production, although this remains to be proven. Soybeans are especially rich in a phytosterol called beta-sitosterol. A 3½-ounce serving of soybeans provides approximately 90 milligrams of beta-sitosterol.

Legumes

In this list, ½ cup of each item, cooked or sprouted, equals 1 serving.

Black-eyed peas

Chickpeas

Garbanzo beans

Kidney beans

Lentils

Lima beans

Pinto beans

Soybeans, including tofu (omit 1 fat serving)

Split peas

Other dried beans and peas

List 5: Fats and Oils

As discussed in Chapters 8 and 10, too much fat in the diet, especially saturated fat, is linked to numerous diseases, including breast cancer, heart disease, and stroke. As you have read, most nutrition experts recommend that you keep total fat intake to below 30% of total calories. They recommend also that you consume at least twice as much unsaturated fat as saturated fat.

Fats and Oils

Each of the following items equals 1 serving.

Mono-unsaturated

Olive oil, 1 teaspoon

Olives, 5 small

Polyunsaturated

Almonds, 10 whole

Avocado (4-inch diameter), 1/8 fruit

Peanuts

    Spanish, 20 whole

    Virginia, 10 whole

Pecans, 2 large

Seeds

    Flax, 1 tablespoon

    Pumpkin, 1 tablespoon

    Sesame, 1 tablespoon

    Sunflower, 1 tablespoon

Vegetable oil

    Canola, 1 teaspoon

    Corn, 1 teaspoon

    Flaxseed, 1 teaspoon

    Safflower, 1 teaspoon

    Soy, 1 teaspoon

    Sunflower, 1 teaspoon

Walnuts, 6 small

Saturated (use sparingly)

Bacon, 1 slice

Butter, 1 teaspoon

Cream, heavy, 1 tablespoon

Cream, light or sour, 2 tablespoons

Cream cheese, 1 tablespoon

Mayonnaise, 1 teaspoon

Salad dressing, 2 teaspoons

List 6: Milk

Is milk for everybody? Definitely not. Many people are allergic to milk or lack the enzymes necessary to digest it. The drinking of cow's milk is a relatively new dietary practice for humans. This may be the reason so many people have difficulty with milk. Milk contains a protein known as casein, which appears to promote atherosclerosis.[7] Many meal-replacement formulas, including Ultra Slim Fast, contain casein. Casein is also used in glues, molded plastics, and paints. Alternatives to cow's milk and casein-containing formulas are soy milk and soy-based formulas. Unlike casein, soy protein actually lowers cholesterol.[8]

Milk

Of each of the following items, 1 cup equals 1 "milk" serving, but for some items you must omit 1 or more fat servings to maintain the nutrition balance of your diet.

Nonfat milk or yogurt

Nonfat soy milk

2% milk or soy milk (omit 1 fat serving)

Lowfat yogurt (omit 1 fat serving)

Whole milk (omit 2 fat servings)

Yogurt (omit 2 fat servings)

List 7: Meats, Fish, Cheese, and Eggs

When choosing from this list, choose primarily from the lowfat group and remove the skin of poultry. This practice will keep the amount of saturated fat low. List 7 provides high concentrations of certain nutrients difficult to get in an entirely vegetarian diet. It provides the full range of amino acids, vitamin B12, and heme iron. The foods in list 7 are sources of nutrients critical to healthy sexual function. Nonetheless, these foods should be eaten in small amounts; 3 or 4 servings daily provide ample amounts of protein and other nutrients.

As you choose from list 7, remember the health-promoting properties of the omega-3 fatty acids in fish oil. Do not use the fact that fish contain these acids as a license to overeat fish, however. Remember that flaxseed oil contains linolenic acid, an omega-3 oil that the body can convert to one of the substances in fish oil. In addition, flaxseed oil also contains lignans, which can reduce the risk of breast cancer.

Meats, Fish, Cheese, and Eggs
Each of the following items equals 1 serving.
Lowfat items
Beef, 1 ounce
    Baby beef, chipped beef, chuck, round (bottom, top), rump (all cuts), spareribs, steak (flank, plate), tenderloin plate ribs, tripe
Cottage cheese, lowfat, ¼ cup
Fish, 1 ounce
Lamb, 1 ounce
    Leg, loin (roast and chops), ribs, shank, shoulder, sirloin
Poultry (chicken or turkey without skin), 1 ounce
Veal, 1 ounce
    Cutlet, leg, loin, rib, shank, shoulder

Medium-fat items
For each of the following items, omit ½ fat serving.
Beef, 1 ounce
    Canned corned beef, ground (15% fat), rib eye, round (ground commercial)

Cheese, 1 ounce

>Farmer, Mozzarella, Parmesan, ricotta

Eggs, 1

Organ meats, 1 ounce

Peanut butter, 2 tablespoons

Pork, 1 ounce

>Boiled, Boston butt, Canadian bacon, loin (all tenderloin), picnic

High-fat items

For each of the following items, omit 2 fat servings.

Beef, 1 ounce

>Brisket, corned beef, ground beef (more than 20% fat), hamburger, roasts (rib), steaks (club and rib)

Cheese, cheddar, 1 ounce

Duck or goose, 1 ounce

Lamb, breast, 1 ounce

Pork, 1 ounce

>Country-style ham, deviled ham, ground pork, loin, spareribs

Menu Planning

The Healthy Exchange System was created to ensure that you are consuming a diet that provides adequate nutrients in their proper ratio. This chapter has given you the number of servings required from each Healthy Exchange List for a 2,500-calorie-a-day diet. These exchange recommendations will help you a great deal in constructing a daily menu—and so will the recipes you will find in the following pages. For more recipes, see my book *The Healing Power of Foods Cookbook*.

Breakfast

Breakfast is an absolute must. Healthful breakfast choices include whole-grain cereals, muffins, and breads, along with fresh whole fruit or fresh fruit juice. Cereals, both hot and cold, and preferably from whole grains, may be the best food choices for breakfast. The complex carbohydrates in the grains provide sustained energy. As mentioned previously, blood cholesterol levels are lowest among adults eating whole-grain cereal for breakfast. Here are a couple of breakfast suggestions.

Granolalike Breakfast

Makes 4 servings

4	cups rolled oats
4	tablespoons sesame seed (ground)
4	tablespoons sunflower seed (ground)
4	tablespoons flaxseed (ground)
¼	cup fresh apple juice
	Cinnamon, to taste
1	cup fresh fruit

In a large bowl, mix oats and ground ingredients. Put ½ cup of oat mixture in a small bowl. Store the bulk of the mixture, covered, in the refrigerator. To the ½ cup of grain mixture, add apple juice and stir. Cover and store overnight in the refrigerator. When ready to serve, add cinnamon and 1 cup fresh fruit to the large bowl; stir. Add the contents of the small bowl; stir and serve.

Dietary Servings Per Recipe Serving
Fruits: 1
Grains and starches: 2
Fats: 3

Nutrition Information Per Recipe Serving
Calories: 350
Carbohydrate: 55%
Protein: 18%
Fat: 27%
Fiber: 1 gram
Calcium: 94 milligrams

Apple-Carrot Muffins

Makes 12 servings (1 muffin per serving)

2½	cups whole-wheat flour
½	cup soy powder
1	teaspoon baking soda
¼	teaspoon salt
¼	teaspoon nutmeg
¼	teaspoon cinnamon
⅛	cup oil
¾	cup raw honey
1	teaspoon vanilla
½	cup apple, grated
½	cup carrot, grated
	Oil, for greasing tin

In a medium-sized bowl, combine all the dry ingredients. In a large bowl, combine all the liquid ingredients. Stir in the apple and carrot. Add the dry ingredients to the liquid mixture. Preheat oven to 400 degrees F. Oil one muffin tin. Spoon the batter into the cups until they are two-thirds full. Bake until a toothpick stuck in the center of a muffin comes out dry (about 20 minutes).

Dietary Servings Per Recipe Serving
Fruits: 1
Grains and starches: 2
Fats: ¹/₈

Nutrition Information Per Recipe Serving:

Calories: 220	Fat: 25%
Carbohydrate: 60%	Fiber: 4 grams
Protein: 15%	Calcium: 53 milligrams

An Apple-Carrot Muffin is a great way to start the day, along with a glass of fresh orange juice.

Lunch

Lunch is a fine time to enjoy a healthful bowl of soup, a large salad, and some whole-grain bread. Bean soups and other legume dishes are especially good lunch selections for people with diabetes and blood sugar problems; these selections can improve blood sugar regulation. Legumes are filling, yet low in calories.

Black-Bean Soup

Makes 4 servings

2	teaspoons extra-virgin olive oil *or* canola oil
2	medium red onions, chopped
1	jalapeño chile, minced
2	large garlic cloves, minced
1	teaspoon ground cumin
½	teaspoon chili powder
2	cups water
4	cups cooked black beans
2	tablespoons sour cream (*optional*)

In a medium saucepan, heat olive oil. Add onion and chile. Cook over moderate heat, stirring frequently, until onion begins to brown (about 4 minutes). Stir in garlic. Reduce heat to low and cook, stirring constantly, for 1 minute. Stir in cumin and chili powder. Remove from heat. In a large heavy pot, place the water, beans, and spice mixture. Cook over low heat, stirring occasionally, until beans are hot (about 5 minutes). If a smooth texture is preferred, transfer the soup to a food processor or blender and purée before serving. Top each serving with sour cream.

Dietary Servings Per Recipe Serving
Vegetables: 1
Legumes: 2
Fats: ½

Nutrition Information Per Recipe Serving
Calories: 248
Carbohydrate: 65%
Protein: 19%
Fat: 16%
Fiber: 22 grams
Calcium: 137 milligrams

This soup can be made up to four days ahead. Simply refrigerate it in an airtight container, then reheat the soup when you're ready.

Herb Dressing

Makes 8 servings (2 tablespoons per serving)

6   tablespoons vegetable oil
2   teaspoons chopped fresh parsley
2   teaspoons chopped fresh chives

2   tablespoons chopped fresh chervil *or* 2 teaspoons
     dried chervil
     Black pepper, to taste
½   cup rice vinegar
2   tablespoons water
3   cloves garlic, minced
2   teaspoons dried mustard

In a blender, combine all ingredients. Blend thoroughly.

Snacks

The best snacks are nuts, seeds, and fresh fruit and vegetables.
If you have a sweet tooth, here is a healthful cookie recipe.

Sunflower Power Cookies

Makes 24 servings (1 cookie per serving)

1   cup chopped dried apricots
     Oil, for greasing pan
¼   cup raw honey
1   tablespoon vegetable oil
1   teaspoon vanilla
2   cups rolled oats
1   cup whole-wheat pastry flour
¼   cup toasted wheat germ
½   cup currants *or* raisins
1   tablespoon sunflower seed
2   tablespoons apple *or* orange juice, if needed

Preheat oven to 350 degrees F. Cover apricots with warm
water; soak them for 15 minutes. Oil a 13- by 9-inch baking
pan. In a large bowl, mix honey, oil, and vanilla. In a medium

bowl, combine oats, flour, and wheat germ. Add flour mixture to wet mixture. Drain apricots. Fold apricots, currants, and sunflower seed into the large bowl, using apple juice to make the batter more pliable if it is too stiff. Press dough into baking pan. Bake for 20 to 25 minutes. Cool and cut into squares.

Dietary Servings Per Recipe Serving
Fruits: 1
Grains and starches: ½
Fats: ¼

Nutrition Information Per Recipe Serving
Calories: 136
Carbohydrate: 66%
Protein: 8%
Fat: 26%
Fiber: 8 grams
Calcium: 75 milligrams

Dinner

For dinner, the most healthful meals contain a fresh vegetable salad, a cooked vegetable side dish or bowl of soup, whole grains, and legumes. The whole grains may be provided in bread, pasta, or pizza; as a side dish; or in an entrée. The legumes can be in soups, salads, and main dishes.

Although a varied diet rich in whole grains, vegetables, and legumes can provide optimal levels of protein, many people like to eat meat. The important thing is not to over-consume animal products. Limit your intake to no more than 4 to 6 ounces per day, and choose fish, skinless poultry, and lean cuts rather than fat-ladened choices.

The next recipe is a great alternative to Beef Stroganoff and provides a complete-protein meal from vegetarian sources.

Mushroom Stroganoff with Tofu

Makes 4 servings

Stroganoff

1	teaspoon canola oil *or* olive oil
½	onion, minced
1	clove garlic, minced (*optional*)
1	pound fresh mushrooms, sliced
4	ounces tofu, cut into 1-inch cubes
1	teaspoon oregano
2	cups cooked brown rice
1	tablespoon toasted slivered almonds
1	tablespoon chopped fresh parsley

Sauce

8	ounces tofu
¼	cup water
2	tablespoons soy sauce
2	tablespoons lemon juice *or* apple cider vinegar
1	clove garlic
1	teaspoon chopped ginger root

Make sauce first. In a large skillet, heat oil. Add onion and garlic; sauté until onion is transparent. Add mushrooms; sauté until they are slightly limp and moisture has evaporated. Remove ingredients from skillet and set them aside. Add tofu cubes to skillet and brown them slightly. Return sautéed ingredients to skillet. Pour sauce over all. Mix well and heat through, stirring. Blend in oregano. Serve over cooked brown rice (½ cup per person) and sprinkle with almonds and parsley.

Sauce   In a blender, combine all ingredients. Blend until very smooth; be sure garlic and ginger root are finely chopped and not left in chunks. Set aside or refrigerate to use later; this improves flavor. Sauce will keep up to one week.

Dietary Servings Per Recipe Serving
Vegetables: ½
Grains and starches: 1
Legumes: 1
Fats: ½

Nutrition Information Per Recipe Serving
Calories: 208
Carbohydrate: 56%
Protein: 21%
Fat: 23%
Fiber: 3 grams
Calcium: 160 milligrams

Final Comments

The dietary guidelines presented in this chapter are designed to provide the menopausal and postmenopausal woman with optimal nutrition. In addition to providing essential nutrients for proper sexual and reproductive function, these dietary recommendations will help maintain healthy bones and reduce the risk of osteoporosis, lower cholesterol levels, and reduce the risk of heart disease and breast cancer.

I firmly believe that the quality of a person's life is directly related to the quality of the foods he or she routinely ingests. The human body is the most remarkable machine in the world, but most Americans are not feeding the body the high-quality fuel it deserves. If you do not feed your body the full range of nutrients it needs, how can it be expected to stay in a state of good health? It can't. Feed your body high-quality fuel, and it will serve you well. Remember: The body is the vessel of the soul. Treat it as your most prized possession.

12

Nutritional
Supplementation

In the last few years, more Americans than ever are taking nutritional supplements. Despite the fact that there is tremendous scientific evidence to support nutritional supplementation, medical experts have not overwhelmingly endorsed it. Some say diet alone can provide all the essential nutrition necessary; many others tout the health benefits of vitamin and mineral supplements. The consumer is left in the middle, trying to figure out which side is right.

First of all, to an extent, both sides are right. What it boils down to is what criteria of "optimal" nutrition are being used. If an expert believes optimal nutrition simply means no obvious signs of nutrient deficiency, his or her answer about whether supplementation is necessary will be different from that of an expert who thinks it means the level of nutrition that allows a person to function at the highest degree, with vitality and enthusiasm for living. What it comes down to, then, is an argument of philosophy.

Do you believe that health is simply a matter of not being sick? Or, do you believe health is much more? It is the goal of optimal health that drives people to take nutritional supplements.

Who Takes Vitamins?

Taking vitamin and mineral supplements has become a way of life for most Americans. Data from the first and second United States Health and Nutrition Examination Survey (HANES I and II), conducted in the 1970s, indicated that almost 35% of the U.S. population between 18 and 74 years of age took vitamin or mineral supplements regularly.[1] During the 1980s and early 1990s, that number has nearly doubled, so that now over 60% of Americans take vitamin or mineral supplements.

Although somewhat outdated, the HANES data demonstrated some interesting facts about supplement users.[1] Perhaps the most interesting finding was that persons with the highest dietary nutrient intakes are the most likely to take a multiple-vitamin, multiple-mineral supplement. This is extremely significant because it says a great deal about how these individuals view "optimal" nutrition. They are not using nutritional supplements to replace a nutrient-poor diet. Instead, they are using supplements as they are intended—that is, to supplement a healthful diet.

The list that follows presents other interesting findings from the HANES studies:

College-educated individuals are much more likely to take a multiple-vitamin, multiple-mineral supplement than those with less education.

More women take supplements than men.

Supplement use is highest in the West and lowest in the South.

Individuals of normal weight or less are more likely to take supplements than heavier individuals.

Individuals who exercise regularly are more likely to take a supplement than those who do not exercise regularly.

The Need for Nutritional Supplementation

Many Americans consume a diet inadequate in nutrition but not so inadequate that nutrient deficiencies are apparent. The term *subclinical deficiency*, or *marginal deficiency*, is often used to describe this state. Complicating this matter is the fact that, in many instances, the only clue of a subclinical nutrient deficiency may be fatigue, lethargy, difficulty in concentration, a lack of a feeling of well-being, or some other vague symptom. Diagnosis of subclinical deficiencies is an extremely difficult process that involves detailed dietary or laboratory analysis.

Is there evidence to support the contention that subclinical vitamin and mineral deficiencies exist? Definitely yes. During recent years the U.S. government has sponsored a number of comprehensive studies (HANES I and II, Ten State Nutrition Survey, USDA nationwide food consumption studies, and so on) to determine the nutrition status of the population. These studies have revealed that marginal nutrient deficiencies exist in approximately 50% of the U.S. population. In addition, the studies showed that, for some selected nutrients in certain age groups, more than 80% of the group consumed less than the recommended dietary allowance (RDA).[2]

These studies indicate that the chance of consuming a diet that meets the RDA for all nutrients is extremely slim for most Americans. In other words, though it is theoretically possible for a healthy individual to get all the nutrition he or she needs from foods, the fact is that most Americans do not even come close to meeting all their nutrition needs through diet alone. In an effort to increase their intake of essential nutrients, many Americans look to vitamin and mineral supplements.

Is the RDA Enough?

The RDAs for vitamins and minerals have been prepared by the Food and Nutrition Board of the National Research Council since 1941.[3] These guidelines were originally developed to reduce the rates of severe nutrition-deficiency diseases, such as scurvy (a deficiency of vitamin C), pellagra (a deficiency of niacin), and beriberi (a deficiency of vitamin B1). Another critical point is that the RDAs were designed to serve as the basis for evaluating the adequacy of diets of groups of people, not individuals. The nutrition requirements of individuals vary widely. As the Food and Nutrition Board put it: "Individuals with special nutritional needs are not covered by the RDAs."

A tremendous amount of scientific research indicates that the optimal level for many nutrients—especially the so-called antioxidant nutrients such as vitamins C and E, beta-carotene, and selenium—may be much higher than their current RDA. To reiterate, the RDAs focus only on the prevention of nutrition deficiencies in population groups, they do not define optimal intake for an individual.

Other factors the RDAs do not adequately take into consideration involve environment and lifestyle. Factors that correspond to environment and lifestyle can destroy vitamins and bind minerals. For example, the Food and Nutrition Board acknowledges that smokers require at least twice as much vitamin C as do nonsmokers.[3] But, what about other nutrients and smoking? And what about the effects of alcohol consumption, food additives, heavy metals (lead, mercury, and the like), carbon monoxide, and other chemicals associated with our modern society? These substances are known to interfere with nutrient function. The need to compensate for the hazards of modern living may be another reason why many people take supplements.

The RDAs have done a good job of defining nutrient intake levels to prevent nutrition deficiencies. In terms of optimum intake of nutrients, however, they are just a starting point.

Guidelines for Vitamin and Mineral Supplementation

There are 13 different known vitamins, each with its own special role to play. The vitamins are classified into two groups: fat-soluble (A, D, E, and K) and water-soluble (the B vitamins and vitamin C). Vitamins function with enzymes in chemical reactions necessary for human bodily function, including energy production. Together, vitamins and enzymes work as catalysts to speed the making or breaking of chemical bonds that join molecules together.

There are 22 different minerals important in human nutrition. Minerals function, along with vitamins, as components of body enzymes. Minerals are also needed for proper composition of bone, blood, and the maintenance of normal cell function.

This book provides many examples of the specific benefits of specific vitamins or minerals. Nutrients interact in the body, however, so the best way to ensure maximum benefit is to provide optimal levels of all essential vitamins and minerals.

Table 12.1 recommends the daily intake of supplemental vitamins and minerals for maintaining the health of menopausal and postmenopausal women. These levels are most easily attained by taking a good multiple-vitamin,

Table 12.1   Optimal Supplementation Range for Women

Supplement Vitamins	Daily Dosage
Vitamin A (retinol)	5,000–10,000 IU*
Vitamin A (from beta-carotene)	10,000–75,000 IU
Vitamin D	100–400 IU
Vitamin E (d-alpha tocopherol)	400–1,200 IU
Vitamin K (phytonadione)	60–900 μg†
Vitamin C (ascorbic acid)	500–3,000 mg
Vitamin B1 (thiamine)	10–90 mg
Vitamin B2 (riboflavin)	10–90 mg
Niacin	10–90 mg
Niacinamide	10–30 mg
Vitamin B6 (pyridoxine)	25–100 mg
Biotin	100–300 μg
Pantothenic acid	25–100 mg
Folic acid	400–1,000 μg
Vitamin B12	400–1,000 μg
Choline	150–500 mg
Inositol	150–500 mg
Minerals	
Boron	3–5 mg
Calcium	250–750 mg
Chromium	200–400 μg
Copper	1–2 mg
Iodine	50–150 μg
Iron	15–30 mg
Magnesium	250–750 mg
Manganese	10–15 mg
Molybdenum	10–25 μg
Potassium	200–500 mg
Selenium	100–200 μg
Silica	200–1,000 μg
Vanadium	50–100 μg
Zinc	15–30 mg

*IU = international units
†μg = microgram (one-millionth of a gram)

multiple-mineral formula and then adding specific nutrients (vitamin C, vitamin E, or calcium, for example) as needed.

Final Comments

The information available at this time indicates that bolstering the diet by taking vitamin and mineral supplements may be of great benefit to menopausal and postmenopausal women. Although individual vitamins and minerals, like vitamin E and calcium, may offer some specific benefits, the goal of nutritional supplementation is to provide a firm foundation. Because the actions of nutrients are interrelated, a broad-spectrum approach offers advantages.

In addition to vitamins and minerals, this book has featured several other nutritional supplements that provide exceptional health benefits to menopausal and postmenopausal women: gamma-oryzanol, bioflavonoids such as hesperidin, and glucosamine sulfate.

13

Design of an Exercise Program

For menopausal and postmenopausal women, the health benefits of regular exercise cannot be overstated. Regular exercise is particularly important in reducing the frequency of hot flashes, maintaining healthy bones, and reducing the risk of heart disease.[1]

The immediate effect of exercise is stress on the body; however, with a regular exercise program the body adapts. The body's response to regular stress is that it becomes stronger, functions more efficiently, and has greater endurance. Exercise is a vital component of health. Figure 13.1 summarizes the benefits of regular exercise.

Physical Benefits of Exercise

The entire body benefits from regular exercise, largely as a result of improved cardiovascular and respiratory function. Simply stated, exercise enhances the transport of oxygen and nutrients into cells. At the same time, exercise enhances

---

Relief from hot flashes

Improved heart function

Improved circulation

Reduced blood pressure

Decreased blood cholesterol levels

Improved ability to deal with stress

Improved oxygen and nutrient utilization in all tissues

Increased self-esteem, mood, and frame of mind

Increased endurance and energy levels

Figure 13.1   The health benefits of regular exercise

the transport of carbon dioxide and waste products from the tissues to the bloodstream and, ultimately, to eliminative organs.

Exercise is particularly important in preventing heart disease. Exercise lowers cholesterol, improves the blood and oxygen supply to the heart, increases the functional capacity of the heart, reduces blood pressure, reduces obesity, and exerts a favorable effect on blood clotting.[2]

Psychological and Social Benefits of Exercise

Regular exercise not only makes people look better, it makes them feel better. Tensions, depressions, feelings of inadequacy, and worries diminish greatly with regular exercise. The value of an exercise program in the treatment of depression cannot be overstated. Exercise alone has been demonstrated to have a tremendous impact on improving mood and the ability to handle stressful life situations. A recent study published in the *American Journal of Epidemiology* revealed that increased participation in exercise, sports, and physical activities is strongly associated with decreased symptoms of depression. These symptoms included feelings that life was not worthwhile, low spirits, anxiety (restlessness and tension), and malaise (feeling run-down, suffering from insomnia, and the like).[3]

How to Start an Exercise Program

The first thing to do before beginning an exercise program is to make sure you are fit enough to start. If you have been mostly inactive for a number of years or have a previously diagnosed illness, see your physician first.

If you are fit enough to begin, the next thing to do is select an activity that you feel you would enjoy. For maximum benefit, the best exercises are the kind that get your heart moving and involve weight bearing. Walking briskly, jogging, cross-country skiing, aerobic dance, and racquet sports are good examples. Although swimming and bicycling are good for your heart, they are not as good for your bones as the weight-bearing exercises.

Brisk walking (4 to 5 miles an hour) for approximately 30 minutes may be the very best form of exercise for weight loss. Walking can be done anywhere; it doesn't require any expensive equipment, just comfortable clothing and well-fitting shoes. And the risk for injury is extremely low. If you are unable to walk outside year-round, join a health club or purchase a treadmill.

Aerobic exercise generally enhances weight-loss programs. Weight training programs can substantially alter body composition by increasing lean body weight and decreasing body fat.[4] Thus, weight training may be just as, or more effective than, aerobic exercise in maintaining or increasing lean body weight.[5] The concept of "spot reduction" is a myth. Exercise draws from all the fat stores of the body, not just from local deposits.

Intensity

Exercise intensity is determined by measuring your heart rate (the number of times your heart beats) per minute. This can be quickly done by placing your index and middle fingers of one hand on the side of the neck, just below the angle of the jaw, or on the opposite wrist. Beginning with zero, count the number of heartbeats for 6 seconds. Simply add a zero to the number of heartbeats and you have your heart rate per minute. For example, if you count 14 beats, your heart rate is 140. Is this a good number? It depends upon your training zone.

The training zone is the rate of exercise that allows you to burn fat, not muscle. The training zone is defined in terms of heart rate per minute. To determine your maximum training heart rate, simply subtract your age from 185. For example, if you are 40 years old, your maximum heart rate is 145. To determine the bottom of the training zone, simply subtract 20 from the maximum rate. If you are 40, this is 125. So, if you are 40 years old, your training range is between 125 and 145 heartbeats per minute. For maximum health benefits, you must stay in this range and never exceed it.

Duration and Frequency

A minimum of 15 to 20 minutes of exercise at your training heart rate at least three times a week is necessary to gain any significant benefits from exercise. It is better to exercise at the lower end of your training zone for longer periods than it is to exercise at a higher intensity for shorter periods. It is also better if you can make exercise a part of your daily routine.

Final Comments

The key to getting the maximum benefit from exercise is to make it enjoyable. Choose an activity that you can have fun with. If you can find enjoyment in exercise, you are much more likely to exercise regularly. You don't get in good physical condition by exercising once, you must do it on a regular basis. So, make it fun and do it often.

References

Chapter 1: Is Estrogen Replacement Therapy Necessary?

1. Wilson RA: Feminine Forever. Evans, New York, 1966.
2. Rubin GL, Peterson HB, Lee NC, et al.: Estrogen replacement therapy and the risk of endometrial cancer: Remaining controversies. Am J Obstet Gynecol 162:148–54, 1990.
3. Whitehead MI, Townsend PT, Davies-Pryse J, et al.: Effects of estrogens and progestins on the biochemistry and morphology of the postmenopausal endometrium. N Engl J Med 305:1599–1685, 1981.
4. Session DR, Kelly AC, and Jewelewicz R: Current concepts in estrogen replacement therapy in the menopause. Fertil Steril 59:277–84, 1993.
5. Birkenfeld A and Kase NG: Menopause medicine: Current treatment options and trends. Compre Ther 17:36–45, 1991.
6. Henrich JB: The postmenopausal estrogen/breast cancer controversy. JAMA 268:1900–2, 1992.
7. Armstrong BK: Oestrogen therapy after the menopause. Boon or bane? Med J Austral 148:213–4, 1988.
8. DuPont WD and Page DL: Menopausal estrogen replacement therapy and breast cancer. Arch Int Med 151:67–72, 1991.
9. Steinberg KK, Thacker SB, Smith SJ, et al.: A meta-analysis of the effect of estrogen replacement therapy on the risk of breast cancer. JAMA 265:1985–90, 1991.

10. Theisen SC and Mansfield PK: Menopause: Social construction or biological destiny. J Health Educ 24:209–13, 1993.
11. Martin MC, Block JE, Sanchez SD, et al.: Menopause without symptoms: The endocrinology of menopause among rural Mayan Indians. Am J Obstet Gynecol 168:1839–45, 1993.

Chapter 2: Hot Flashes

1. Hammar M, Berg G, and Lindgren R: Does physical exercise influence the frequency of postmenopausal hot flushes? Acta Obstet Gynecol Scand 69:409–12, 1990.
2. Albert-Puleo M: Fennel and anise as estrogenic agents. J Ethnopharmacol 2:337–44, 1980.
3. Kaldas RS and Hughes CL: Reproductive and general metabolic effects of phytoestrogens in mammals. Reprod Toxicol 3:81–9, 1989.
4. Christy CJ: Vitamin E in menopause. Am J Obstet Gynecol 50:84–7, 1945.
5. McLaren HC: Vitamin E in the menopause. Br Med J ii:1378–81, 1949.
6. Finkler RS: The effect of vitamin E in the menopause. J Clin Endocrinol Metab 9:89–94, 1949.
7. Smith CJ: Non-hormonal control of vasomotor flushing in menopausal patients. Chic Med 67:193–5, 1964.
8. Murase Y and Iishima H: Clinical studies of oral administration of gamma-oryzanol on climacteric complaints and its syndrome. Obstet Gynecol Prac 12:147–9, 1963.
9. Ishihara M: Effect of gamma-oryzanol on serum lipid peroxide levels and climacteric disturbances. Asia Oceania J Obstet Gynecol 10:317, 1984.
10. Yoshino G, Kazumi T, Amano M, et al.: Effects of gamma-oryzanol on hyperlipidemic subjects. Current Ther Res 45:543–52, 1989.
11. Rose DP: Dietary fiber, phytoestrogens, and breast cancer. Nutr 8:47–51, 1992.
12. Adlercreutz H, Fotsis T, Bannwart C, et al.: Determination of urinary lignans and phytoestrogen metabolites, potential antiestrogens and anticarcinogens, in urine of women on various habitual diets. Steroid Biochem 25:791–7, 1986.
13. Elghamry MI and Shihata IM: Biological activity of phytoestrogens. Planta Medica 13:352–7, 1965.

14. Tamaya T, et al.: Inhibition by plant herb extracts of steroid bindings in uterus, liver, and serum of the rabbit. Acta Obstet Gynecol Scand 65:839–42, 1986.

15. Harada M, Suzuki M, and Ozaki Y: Effect of Japanese angelica root and peony root on uterine contraction in the rabbit in situ. J Pharm Dyn 7:304–11, 1984.

16. Yoshiro K: The physiological actions of tang-kuei and cnidium. Bull Oriental Healing Arts Inst USA 10:269–78, 1985.

17. Thastrup O, Fjalland B, and Lemmich J: Coronary vasodilatory, spasmolytic and cAMP-phosphodiesterase inhibitory properties of dihydropyranocoumarins and dihydrofuranocoumarins. Acta Pharmacol Toxicol 52:246–53, 1983.

18. Costello CH and Lynn EV: Estrogenic substances from plants: *I. glycyrrhiza*. J Am Pharm Soc 39:177–80, 1950.

19. Kumagai A, Nishino K, Shimomura A, et al.: Effect of glycyrrhizin on estrogen action. Endocrinol Japan 14:34–8, 1967.

20. Haller J: Animal experimentation with the Lipshutz technique on the activity of a phytohormone on gonadotropin function. Geburt Frauen 18:1347, 1958.

21. Duker EM, Kopanski L, Jarry H, et al.: Effects of extracts from *Cimicifuga racemosa* on gonadotropin release in menopausal women and ovariectomized rats. Planta Medica 57:420–4, 1991.

Chapter 3: Atrophic Vaginitis

1. Ant M: Diabetic vulvovaginitis treated with vitamin E suppositories. Am J Ob Gyn 67:407–10, 1954.

2. Werbach M: Healing Through Nutrition. Harper Collins, New York, NY, 1993, pp. 247–8.

3. McLaren HC: Vitamin E in the menopause. Br Med J ii:1378–81, 1949.

4. Messina M and Barnes S: The roles of soy products in reducing risk of cancer. J Natl Cancer Inst 83:541–6, 1991.

5. Messina M and Messina V: Increasing the use of soyfoods and their potential role in cancer prevention. J Am Diet Assoc 91:836–40, 1991.

Chapter 4: Bladder Infections

1. Marshall FF and Middleton AW: Eosinophilic cystitis. J Urol 112: 225–8, 1974.

2. Goldstein M: Eosinophilic cystitis. J Urol 106:854–7, 1972.

3. Palacios AS, Juana AD, Sagarra JM, and Duque RA: Eosinophilic food-induced cystitis. Allergol et Immunopathol 12:463–9, 1984.

4. Prodromos PN, Brusch CA, and Ceresia GC: Cranberry juice in the treatment of urinary tract infections. Southwest Med 47:17, 1968.

5. Sternlieb P: Cranberry juice in renal disease. N Engl J Med 268:57, 1963.

6. Moen DV: Observations on the effectiveness of cranberry juice in urinary infections. Wisconsin Med J 61:282, 1962.

7. Kahn DH, Panariello VA, Saeli J, et al.: Effect of cranberry juice on urine. J Am Dietetic Assoc 51:251, 1967.

8. Bodel PT, Cotran R, and Kass EH: Cranberry juice and the antibacterial action of hippuric acid. J Lab Clin Med 54:881, 1959.

9. Sobota AE: Inhibition of bacterial adherence by cranberry juice: Potential use for the treatment of urinary tract infections. J Urol 131:1013–6, 1984.

10. Ofek I, Goldhar J, et al.: Anti-*escherichia* activity of cranberry and blueberry juices. N Engl J Med 324:1599, 1991.

11. Sanchez A, Reeser J, Lau H, et al.: Role of sugars in human neutrophilic phagocytosis. Am J Clin Nutr 26:1180–4, 1973.

12. Bernstein J, Alpert S, Nauss K, and Suskind R: Depression of lymphocyte transformation following oral glucose ingestion. Am J Clin Nutr 30:613, 1977.

13. Munday PE and Savage S: Cymalon in the management of urinary tract symptoms. Genitourin Med 66:461, 1990.

14. Spooner JB: Alkalinization in the management of cystitis. J Int Med Res 12:30–4, 1984.

15. Merck Index, 10th edition. Merck & Company, Rahway, NJ, 1983, pp. 112–3, 699.

16. Frohne V: Untersuchungen zur frage der harndesifizierenden wirkungen von barentraubenblatt-extracten. Planta Medica 18:1–25, 1970.

17. Leung A: Encyclopedia of Common Natural Ingredients Used in Food, Drugs, and Cosmetics. Wiley, New York, 1980.

18. Amin AH, Subbaiah TV, and Abbasi KM: Berberine sulfate: Antimicrobial activity, bioassay, and mode of action. Can J Microbiol 15:1067–76, 1969.

19. Reid G, Bruce AW, and Cook RL: Effect on urogenital flora of antibiotic therapy for urinary tract infection. Scand J Infect Dis 22:43–7, 1990.

20. Lidefelt KJ, Bollgren I, and Nord CE: Changes in periurethral micro-flora after antimicrobial drugs. Arch Dis Child 66:683–5, 1991.

Chapter 5: Cold Hands and Feet

1. Barnes BO and Galton L: Hypothyroidism: The Unsuspected Illness. Thomas Crowell, New York, NY, 1976.
2. Langer SE and Scheer JF: Solved: The Riddle of Illness. Keats, New Canaan, CT, 1984.
3. Jacobs AM and Owen GM: The effect of age on iron absorption. J Gerontol 24:95–6, 1969.
4. Viteri FE and Torun B: Anaemia and physical work capacity. Clin Haematol 3:609–26, 1974.
5. Gardner GW, Edgerton VR, Senewiratne B, et al.: Physical work capacity and metabolic stress in subjects with iron deficiency anemia. Am J Clin Nutr 30:910–7, 1977.
6. Fairbanks VF and Beutler E: Iron. In: Modern Nutrition in Health and Disease, 7th edition. Shils ME and Young VR (eds). Lea and Febiger, Philadelphia, 1988, pp. 193–226.
7. Bezwoda W, Charlton R, Bothwell T, et al.: The importance of gastric hydrochloric acid in the absorption of nonheme iron. J Lab Clin Med 92:108–16, 1978.
8. Kleijnen J and Knipschild P: Drug Profiles—*Ginkgo biloba*. Lancet 340:1136–9, 1993.
9. Bauer U: Six-month double-blind randomized clinical trial of *Ginkgo biloba* extract versus placebo in two parallel groups in patients suffering from peripheral arterial insufficiency. Arzneim-Forsch 34:716–21, 1984.
10. Rudofsky VG: The effect of *Ginkgo biloba* extract in cases of arterial occlusive disease—A randomized placebo controlled double-blind cross-over study. Fortschr Med 105:397–400, 1987.

Chapter 6: Forgetfulness, Mental Distractedness, and Depression

1. Brown MB (ed): Present Knowledge in Nutrition, 6th edition. Nutrition Foundation, Washington, DC, 1990.
2. Werbach MR: Nutritional Influences and Mental Health. Third Line Press, Tarzana, CA, 1991.

3. Kleijnen J and Knipschild P: *Ginkgo biloba* for cerebral insufficiency. Br J Clin Pharmacol 34:352–8, 1992.

4. Kleijnen J and Knipschild P: Drug profiles—*Ginkgo biloba*. Lancet 340:1136–9, 1993.

5. Vorberg G: *Ginkgo biloba* extract (GBE): A long-term study of chronic cerebral insufficiency in geriatric patients. Clin Trials J 22:149–57, 1985.

6. Hofferberth B: Effect of *Ginkgo biloba* extract on neurophysiological and psychometric measurement in patients with cerebroorganic syndrome—A double-blind study versus placebo. Arzneim-Forsch 39:918–22, 1989.

7. Gessner B, Voelp A, and Klasser M: Study of the long-term action of a *Ginkgo biloba* extract on vigilance and mental performance as determined by means of quantitative pharmaco-EEG and psychometric measurements. Arzneim-Forsch 35:1459–65, 1985.

8. Hindmarch I and Subhan Z: The psychopharmacological effects of *Ginkgo biloba* extract in normal healthy volunteers. Int J Clin Pharmacol Res 4:89–93, 1984.

9. Hobbs C: St. John's wort, *Hypericum perforatum*. HerbalGram 18/19:24–33, 1989.

10. Proceedings from The Fourth International Congress on Phytotherapy, Munich, Germany, September 10–13, 1992.

Chapter 7: Maintenance of Healthy Bones

1. Dempster DW and Lindsay R: Pathogenesis of osteoporosis. Lancet 341:797–805, 1993.

2. Grossman M, Kirsner J, and Gillespie I: Basal and histalog-stimulated gastric secretion in control subjects and in patients with peptic ulcer or gastric cancer. Gastroenterol 45:15–26, 1963.

3. Recker R: Calcium absorption and achlorhydria. N Engl J Med 313:70–3, 1985.

4. Nicar MJ and Pak CYC: Calcium bioavailability from calcium carbonate and calcium citrate. J Clin Endocrinol Metabol 61:391–3, 1985.

5. Lore F, Nuti R, Vattimo A, and Caniggia: Vitamin D metabolites in postmenopausal osteoporosis. Horm Metab Res 16:58, 1984.

6. Gallagher J, Riggs L, Eisman J, et al.: Intestinal calcium absorption and serum vitamin D metabolites in normal subjects and osteoporotic patients: Effect of age and dietary calcium. J Clin Invest 64:729–36, 1979.

7. Brautbar N: Osteoporosis: Is 1,25-$(OH)_2D_3$ of value in treatment? Nephron 44:161–6, 1986.

8. Ellis F, Holesh S, and Ellis J: Incidence of osteoporosis in vegetarians and omnivores. Am J Clin Nutr 25:55–8, 1972.

9. Marsh A, Sanchez T, Chaffe F, et al.: Bone mineral mass in adult lactoovovegetarian and omnivorous adults. Am J Clin Nutr 37: 453–6, 1983.

10. Licata A, Bou E, Bartter F, and West F: Acute effects of dietary protein on calcium metabolism in patients with osteoporosis. J Gerontol 36:14–9, 1981.

11. Thom J, Morris J, Bishop A, and Blacklock: The influence of refined carbohydrate on urinary calcium excretion. Br J Urol 50: 459–64, 1978.

12. Bitensky L, Hart JP, Catterall A, et al.: Circulating vitamin K levels in patients with fractures. J Bone Joint Surg 70–B:663–4, 1988.

13. Neilsen FH, Hunt CD, Mullen LM, and Hunt JR: Effect of dietary boron on mineral, estrogen, and testosterone metabolism in postmenopausal women. FASEB J 1:394–7, 1987.

14. Block G: Dietary guidelines and the results of food consumption surveys. Am J Clin Nutr 53:356S–7S, 1991.

15. Nielsen FH, Gallagher SK, Johnson LK, and Nielsen EJ: Boron enhances and mimics some of the effects of estrogen therapy in postmenopausal women. J Trace Elem Exp Med 5:237–46, 1992.

16. Lee CJ, Lawler GS, and Johnson GH: Effects of supplementation of the diets with calcium and calcium-rich foods on bone density of elderly females with osteoporosis. Am J Clin Nutr 34:819–23, 1981.

17. Gaby AR: Preventing and Reversing Osteoporosis. Prima, Rocklin, CA, 1994.

18. Gaby, AR: Preventing and Reversing Osteoporosis. Prima, Rocklin, CA, 1994.

19. Pak CYC and Fuller C: Idiopathic hypocitraturic calcium-oxalate nephrolithiasis successfully treated with potassium citrate. Ann Int Med 104:33–7, 1986.

20. Johansson G, Backman U, Danielson B, et al.: Biochemical and clinical effects of the prophylactic treatment of renal calcium stones with magnesium hydroxide. J Urol 124:770–4, 1980.

21. Cohen L and Kitzes R: Infrared spectroscopy and magnesium content of bone mineral in osteoporotic women. Isr J Med Sci 17:1123–5, 1981.

22. Rude RK, Adams JS, Ryzen E, et al.: Low serum concentration of 1,25-dihydroxyvitamin D in human magnesium deficiency. J Clin Endocrinol Metab 61:933–40, 1985.

23. Seelig MS: Magnesium deficiency with phosphate and vitamin D excess: Role in pediatric cardiovascular nutrition. Cardio Med 3:637–50, 1978.

24. Newcomer A, Hodgson S, McGill D, and Thomas P: Lactase deficiency: Prevalence in osteoporosis. Ann Int Med 89:218–20, 1978.

25. Brattstrom LE, Hultberg BL, and Hardebo JE: Folic acid responsive postmenopausal homocysteinemia. Metab 34:1073–7, 1985.

26. Aloia JF, Cohn SH, Vaswani A, et al.: Risk factors for postmenopausal osteoporosis. Am J Med 78:95–100, 1985.

27. Pocock NA, Eisman JA, Yeates MG, et al.: Physical fitness is the major determinant of femoral neck and lumbar spine density. J Clin Invest 78:618–21, 1986.

28. Krolner B, Toft B, Nielsen S, and Tondevold E: Physical exercise as prophylaxis against involutional vertebral bone loss: A controlled trial. Clin Sci 64:541–6, 1983.

29. Yeater R and Martin R: Senile osteoporosis: The effects of exercise. Postgrad Med 75:147–9, 1984.

30. Marcus R, Drinkwater B, Dalsky G, et al.: Osteoporosis and exercise in women. Med Sci Sports Exer 24:S301–7, 1992.

31. Donaldson C, Hulley S, Vogel J, et al.: Effect of prolonged bed rest on bone mineral. Metab 19:1071–84, 1970.

Chapter 8: Prevention of Breast Cancer

1. National Research Council: Diet and Health. Implications for Reducing Chronic Disease Risk. National Academy Press, Washington, DC, 1989.

2. Rogers AE and Longnecker MP: Biology of disease: Dietary and nutritional influences on cancer: A review of epidemiologic and experimental data. Lab Invest 59:729–59, 1988.

3. Howe GR, Hirohata T, Hislop TG, et al.: Dietary factors and the risk of breast cancer: Combined analysis of 12 case-control studies. J Natl Cancer Inst 82:56–9, 1990.

4. Cohen LA, Rose DP, and Wynder EL: A rationale for dietary intervention in postmenopausal breast cancer patients: An update. Nutr Cancer 19:1–10, 1993.

5. Serraino M and Thompson LU: The effect of flaxseed supplementation on early risk markers for mammary carcinogenesis. Cancer Letters 60:135–42, 1991.

6. Adlercreutz H, Fotsis T, Bannwart C, et al.: Determination of urinary lignans and phytoestrogen metabolites, potential antiestrogens and anticarcinogens, in urine of women in various habitual diets. J Steroid Biochem 25:791–7, 1986.

7. Simpoulos AP: Summary of the NATO Advanced Research Workshop on Dietary μ3 and μ6 fatty acids: Biological effects and nutritional essentiality. J Nutr Med 119:521–8, 1989.

8. Enig MG: Dietary fats and cancer trends—A critique. Fed Proc 37:2215–20, 1978.

9. Mensink RP and Katan MB: Effect of dietary trans fatty acids on high-density and low-density lipoprotein cholesterol levels in health subjects. N Engl J Med 323:439–45, 1990.

10. Steinmetz KA and Potter JD: Vegetables, fruit, and cancer. I. Epidemiology. Cancer Causes Control 2:325–57, 1991.

11. Steinmetz KA and Potter JD: Vegetables, fruit, and cancer. II. Mechanisms. Cancer Causes Control 2:427–42, 1991.

12. Olson JA: Chapter 11: Vitamin A. In: Present Knowledge in Nutrition, 6th edition. Brown MB (ed). Nutrition Foundation, Washington, DC, 1990, pp. 96–107.

13. Bendich A and Olson JA: Biological actions of carotenoids. FASEB J 3:1927–32, 1989.

14. Bendich A: Carotenoids and the immune response. J Nutr Med 119:112–5, 1989.

15. Bendich A: The safety of beta-carotene. Nutr Cancer 11:207–14, 1988.

16. Micozzi MS, Beecher GR, Taylor PR, and Khachik F: Carotenoid analysis of selected raw and cooked foods associated with a lower risk for cancer. J Natl Cancer Inst 82:282–5, 1990.

17. American Cancer Society. Nutrition and Cancer: Cause and Prevention. American Cancer Society, New York, 1984.

18. Petrakis NL and King EB: Cytological abnormalities in nipple aspirates of breast fluid from women with severe constipation. Lancet 2:1203–5, 1981.

19. Hentges DJ: Does diet influence human fecal microflora composition? Nutr Rev 38:329–6, 1980.

20. Aldercreutz H: Diet and breast cancer. Acta Oncol 31:175–81, 1992.

21. Rose DP: Dietary fiber, phytoestrogens, and breast cancer. Nutr 8:47–51, 1992.

22. Goldin B, Aldercreutz H, Dwyer J, et al.: Effect of diet on excretion of estrogens in pre- and postmenopausal women. Cancer Res 41:3771–3, 1981.

23. Messina M and Barnes S: The roles of soy products in reducing risk of cancer. J Natl Cancer Inst 83:541–6, 1991.

24. Messina M and Messina V: Increasing the use of soyfoods and their potential role in cancer prevention. J Am Dietetic Assoc 91:836–40, 1991.

25. Dausch JG and Nixon DW: Garlic: A review of its relationship to malignant disease. Preventive Med 19:346–61, 1990.

26. Ip C, Lisk DJ, and Stoewsanc GS: Mammary cancer prevention by regular garlic and selenium-enriched garlic. Nutr Cancer 17:279–86, 1992.

27. Falck F, Ricci A, Wolff MS, et al.: Pesticides and polychlorinated biphenyl residues in human breast lipids and their relation to breast cancer. Arch Environ Health 47:143–6, 1992.

28. Quillin P: Safe Eating. Evans, New York, 1990.

29. Fan AM and Jackson RJ: Pesticides and food safety. Regulatory Toxicol Pharmacol 9:158–74, 1989.

30. Sterling T and Arundel AV: Health effects of phenoxy herbicides. Scand J Work Environ Health 12:161–73, 1986.

31. Mott L and Broad M: Pesticides in Food. National Resources Defense Council, San Francisco, 1984.

Chapter 9: Relief of Osteoarthritis

1. Murray MT and Pizzorno JE: Encyclopedia of Natural Medicine. Prima, Rocklin, CA, 1990.

2. Bland JH and Cooper SM: Osteoarthritis: A review of the cell biology involved and evidence for reversibility. Management rationally related to known genesis and pathophysiology. Semin Arthr Rheum 14:106–33, 1984.

3. Brooks PM, Potter SR, and Buchanan WW: NSAID and osteo-arthritis—help or hindrance. J Rheumatol 9:3–5, 1982.

4. Shield MJ: Anti-inflammatory drugs and their effects on cartilage synthesis and renal function. Eur J Rheum Inflam 13:7–16, 1993.

5. Perry GH, Smith MJG, and Whiteside CG: Spontaneous recovery of the hip joint space in degenerative hip disease. Ann Rheum Dis 31:440–8, 1972.

6. Newman NM and Ling, RSM: Acetabular bone destruction related to non-steroidal anti-inflammatory drugs. Lancet ii:11–13, 1985.

7. Solomon L: Drug induced arthropathy and necrosis of the femoral head. J Bone Joint Surg 55B:246–51, 1973.

8. Ronningen H and Langeland N: Indomethacin treatment in osteoarthritis of the hip joint. Acta Orthop Scand 50:169–74, 1979.

9. Sullivan MX and Hess WC: Cystine content of finger nails in arthritis. J Bone Joint Surg 16:185–8, 1935.

10. Senturia BD: Results of treatment of chronic arthritis and rheumatoid conditions with colloidal sulphur. J Bone Joint Surg 16: 119–25, 1934.

11. Childers NF: A Diet to Stop Arthritis. Somerset Press, Somerville, NJ, 1991.

12. Vaz AL: Double-blind clinical evaluation of the relative efficacy of ibuprofen and glucosamine sulfate in the management of osteoarthrosis of the knee in out-patients. Current Med Res Opin 8:145–9, 1982.

13. Crolle G and D'este E: Glucosamine sulfate for the management of arthrosis: A controlled clinical investigation. Current Med Res Opin 7:104–14, 1982.

14. Tapadinhas MJ, Rivera IC, and Bignamini AA: Oral glucosamine sulfate in the management of arthrosis: Report on a multi-centre open investigation in Portugal. Pharmatherapeutica 3:157–68, 1982.

15. D'Ambrosia ED, Casa B, Bompani R, et al.: Glucosamine sulphate: A controlled clinical investigation in arthrosis. Pharmatherapeutica 2:504–8, 1982.

Chapter 10: Prevention of Heart Disease

1. National Research Council: Diet and Health. Implications for Reducing Chronic Disease Risk. National Academy Press, Washington, DC, 1989.

2. Wilson PWF: High-density lipoprotein, low-density lipoprotein and coronary artery disease. Am J Cardiol 66:7A–10A, 1990.

3. Schauss A: Dietary Fish Oil Consumption and Fish Oil Supplementation. In: A Textbook of Natural Medicine. Pizzorno JE and Murray MT (eds). Bastyr College Publications, Seattle, 1991. pp. V:Fish Oils:1–7.

4. Von Schacky C: Prophylaxis of atherosclerosis with marine omega-3 fatty acids. A comprehensive strategy. Ann Int Med 107:890–9, 1987.

5. Cobias L, Clifton PS, Abbey M, et al.: Lipid, lipoprotein, and hemostatic effects of fish vs. fishoil μ-3 fatty acids in mildly hyperlipidemic males. Am J Clin Nutr 53:1210–6, 1991.

6. Fraser GE, Sabaté J, Beeson WL, and Strahan TM: A possible protective effect of nut consumption on risk of coronary heart disease. Arch Int Med 152:1416–24, 1992.

7. Robertson J, Brydon WG, Tadesse K, et al.: The effect of raw carrot on serum lipids and colon function. Am J Clin Nutr 32:1889–92, 1979.

8. Stanto JL and Keast DR: Serum cholesterol, fat intake, and breakfast consumption in the United States adult population. J Am Coll Nutr 8:567–72, 1989.

9. Ripsin CM, Keenan JM, Jacobs DR, et al.: Oat products and lipid lowering, a meta-analysis. JAMA 267:3317–25, 1992.

10. Cerda J, Robbins FL, Burgin CW, et al.: The effects of grapefruit pectin on patients at risk for coronary heart disease without altering diet or lifestyle. Clin Cardiol 11:589–94, 1988.

11. Ornish D, Brown SE, Scherwitz LW, et al.: Can lifestyle changes reverse coronary heart disease. Lancet 336:129–33, 1990.

12. Resnicow K, Barone J, Engle A, et al.: Diet and serum lipids in vegan vegetarians: A model for risk reduction. J Am Dietetic Assoc 91:447–53, 1991.

13. The Expert Panel: Report of the National Cholesterol Education Program Expert Panel on detection, evaluation, and treatment of high cholesterol in adults. Arch Int Med 148:136–69, 1988.

14. Canner PL and the Coronary Drug Project Group: Mortality in Coronary Drug Project patients during a nine-year post-treatment period. J Am Coll Cardiol 8:1245–55, 1986.

15. Welsh AL and Ede M: Inositol hexanicotinate for improved nicotinic acid therapy. Int Rec Med 174:9–15, 1961.

16. El-Enein AMA, Hafez YS, Salem H, and Abdel M: The role of nicotinic acid and inositol hexaniacinate as anticholesterolemic and anti-lipemic agents. Nutr Rep Int 28:899–911, 1983.

17. Sunderland GT, Belch JJF, Sturrock RD, et al.: A double blind randomised placebo controlled trial of hexopal in primary Raynaud's disease. Clin Rheumatol 7:46–9, 1988.

Chapter 11: Dietary Guidelines

1. Trowell H, Burkitt D, and Heaton K: Dietary Fibre, Fibre-Depleted Foods and Disease. Academic Press, New York, 1985.

2. US Dept of Health and Human Services: The Surgeon General's Report on Nutrition and Health. Prima, Rocklin, CA, 1988.

3. National Research Council: Diet and Health. Implications for Reducing Chronic Disease Risk. National Academy Press, Washington, DC, 1989.

4. Cheng KK: Pickled vegetables in the aetiology of oesophageal cancer in Hong Kong Chinese. Lancet 339:1314–8, 1992.

5. Tilvis RS and Miettinen TA: Serum plant sterols and their relation to cholesterol absorption. Am J Clin Nutr 43:92–7, 1986.

6. Messina M and Barnes S: The roles of soy products in reducing risk of cancer. J Natl Cancer Inst 83:541–6, 1991.

7. Beynen AC, Van der Meer R, and West CE: Mechanism of casein-induced hypercholesterolemia: Primary and secondary features. Atherosclerosis 60:291–3, 1986.

8. Carrol KK: Review of clinical studies on cholesterol-lowering response to soy protein. J Am Dietetic Assoc 91:820–7, 1991.

Chapter 12: Nutritional Supplementation

1. Block G, Cox C, Madans J, et al.: Vitamin supplement use, by demographic characteristics. Am J Epidemiol 127:297–309, 1988.

2. National Research Council: Diet and Health. Implications for Reducing Chronic Disease Risk. National Academy Press, Washington, DC, 1989.

3. National Research Council: Recommended Dietary Allowances, 10th edition. National Academy Press, Washington, DC, 1989.

Chapter 13: Design of an Exercise Program

1. Shangold MM: Exercise in the menopausal woman. Obstet Gynecol 75:53S–58S, 1990.

2. Pollack ML, Wilmore JH, and Fox SM: Exercise in Health and Disease. Saunders, Philadelphia, 1984.

3. Farmer ME, Locke BZ, Mosciki EK, et al.: Physical activity and depressive symptomatology: The NHANES 1 epidemiologic follow-up study. Am J Epidemiol 1328:1340–51, 1988.

4. Wilmore JH: Alterations in strength, body composition, and athropometric measurements consequent to a 10-week weight training program. Med Sci Sports Exer 6:133–8, 1974.

5. Ballor DL, Katch VL, Becque MD, and Marks CR: Resistance weight training during calorie restriction enhances lean body weight maintenance. Am J Clin Nutr 47:19–25, 1988.

Index